Help! I Can't P

A Guide To Managing Constipation

Helen Irwin

Copyright

Disclaimer

Always consult a qualified medical professional for individual advice before following any new diet or health program and any symptoms that develop while applying the information in this document. The author cannot be held responsible for any loss or claim arising out of the use, or misuse, of the information given or the failure to take medical advice.

Acknowledgements

Thanks to Tony, my husband, for reading early drafts, giving me good constructive feedback, and helping me format my book for publishing.

Thanks to Tony, my son, for editing early drafts and suggesting I include more of my story with the Fact Files.

Thanks to Muhammad Ronnie, my brother, for the drawing of the Colon and Small Intestines.

Thanks to my writing group buddies Susan and Martha for their encouragement and Susan for her help with editing.

Table of Contents

Notes for the Reader

WORD CHOICE AND SPELLING

- The words *colon, large bowel,* and *large intestines* are interchangeable. For clarity, throughout the book, *colon* is used.
- In the US, flatulence is known as *gas*; in the UK, it's more commonly known as *wind.* However, the terminology used in gut testing in the UK is *gas,* so for this book, *gas* is used for flatulence.
- Gut bacteria are considered *good* or *bad,* although sometimes referred to as beneficial or harmful. For consistency, good and bad are used.

REFERENCES

There are no references for the information throughout the book; however, it can be checked by searching the Web for relevant words such as *high-fibre food* or *statistics for constipation.* In addition, included are some links to Websites, YouTube and Facebook.

TITBITS

At the end of each *Fact File* and *My Story*, there is a *Titbit,* a small piece of interesting information often to do with pooping but sometimes not. Here's an index of the *Titbits.*

The Colon and Small Intestines

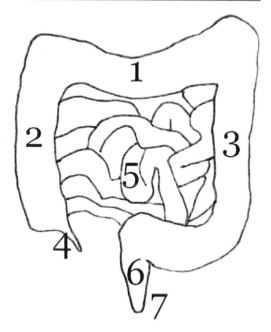

1 Transverse Colon
2 Ascending Colon
3 Descending Colon
4 Appendix
5 Small Intestines
6 Rectum
7 Anus

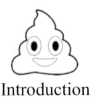

Introduction

Over the years, I've learned things that have given me relief from some of the discomforts of constipation. I've written this book hoping that it may help others find relief. I don't offer a cure as I haven't found one. I simply write about my journey with constipation and how I manage it. I'm not a medical professional but an ordinary woman who has suffered from constipation for over sixty years. Everything I've written is based on my experience and on information I've read or heard from various sources.

Suppose your constipation is acute (short term) rather than chronic (long term). In that case, you may find that you'll quickly correct or manage your constipation by applying some of the information in this book.

Or perhaps you have long-term chronic constipation. You may, like me, have read many books on constipation or viewed some of the thousands of videos on YouTube that promise *if you follow these steps, you'll be pooping regularly in no time.* And, like me, you followed the steps, but regular pooping didn't happen. Or you've taken the advice of people who fixed their constipation with different remedies. For example, drinking three litres of water a day, but when you tried this, it only made visits to the bathroom more frequent. Or switching to a vegan or plant-based diet, but for you, the increase in fibre only caused excessive gas and bloating.

Over many years of looking for ways to find relief, I've learned that our bodies are all different, and what works for one person may not work for another. It's often a combination of practices rather than one practice that helps.

The book's nine chapters each have a *Fact File* and a *My Story*. The *Fact Files* give information on the chapter topic, such as dietary fibre, water, probiotics, and gut tests. These correspond to *My Story*, where I share my experience of applying the *Fact Files* information to manage constipation. You'll read how my constipation began in childhood and then, in recent years, worsened after following a low-carb diet for a year. At the end of the book, there's an Epilogue that sums up my journey.

I've also included an amalgamation of *My Story* from the nine chapters. I did this as I thought you might like to read it through without reading the Fact Files. The chapters are of varying lengths. For example, Chapter 3, *Water* is the shortest, and Chapter 6, *Enemas* is the longest. The size of the chapter depended on how much knowledge and experience I had on each chapter topic.

You'll notice when reading my book that I don't mention visiting doctors or gastroenterologists (gut specialists). When I saw medical professionals, I was only ever prescribed laxatives for my constipation. Sometimes they worked, sometimes they didn't work and frequently caused stomach upsets. However, I'm not against doctors. I have an autoimmune disease and visit doctors and hospitals, take regular medication, and have had knee surgery. I prefer to go for natural remedies for my gut, but that's a decision based on my symptoms, and I'm not recommending this to others.

I also don't write about the use of laxatives for constipation. I'm not against using them; it's just my choice not to use them. However, I do take fibre supplements and use enemas. If you'd like advice and support on laxatives and to read others' experiences of taking them, join the Facebook Support Group – *Chronic Constipation Support | Reversing Chronic Constipation Naturally.*

In recent years I've learned a lot about gut health, and when writing, I considered giving more information, such as on the microbiome. Still, I resisted this, feeling it may distract from the book's topic of constipation. However, you may wish to do further research yourself.

Your journey with constipation may differ from mine; you may have experienced minor or severe symptoms. You may have read widely on the subject or are new to reading about it. A friend who worked as a high school teacher told me that even though he knew his pupils had been taught the basics of a subject in previous years, he taught them again. He said this approach helped fill in any gaps in knowledge before he moved on to the topics for that year.

I've written this book with that approach in mind, starting with the basics, writing about the causes of constipation and how things like an increase of fibre and water can help. However, later in the book, I move past the basics and write about the microbiome, gut testing, and how probiotics and prebiotics in food and supplements benefit our guts. So regardless of your knowledge about constipation, I hope you'll learn something new to help you on your journey.

Best wishes

Helen

1 Constipation

Fact File: Constipation

There's a YouTube video titled 'Making Poop Great Again' by Jackson Long. He believes *publicly discussing our bowel habits is one of the greatest taboos within our society*. A UK survey on *embarrassing things to discuss with your doctor* revealed that bowel health came second to sexually transmitted diseases. We may think it's *only me* when it comes to constipation because no one is talking about it, but this isn't the case.

If you search for *constipation* on the Web, there are over one hundred and thirty million results. Here are a few interesting facts about constipation I read in my Web search.

o The two most common types of constipation are CIC for Chronic Idiopathic Constipation (cause unknown) and IBS-C for Irritable Bowel Syndrome with Constipation.

o Two groups of people suffer more from constipation: the elderly over sixty-five and women, who are up to three times more constipated than men. However, women do live longer than men and that could be part of the reason for these differences.

o The percentage of people who suffer from constipation in the UK and US at any time is 15% to 20%.

STATISTICS ON CONSTIPATION

o The UK has a population of 68 million meaning 9 to 13 million Brits are constipated.

Over 65,000 yearly hospital admissions cost the health service £145 million.

The cost of prescription laxatives is over £1 million annually, which doesn't include laxatives bought over the counter.

o The US has a population of 332 million meaning 48 to 64 million Americans are constipated.

Every year, 2.5 million people visit their doctor for constipation. Annual sales for over-the-counter laxatives add up to £600 million.

Treatment of constipation costs the health care system £180 million annually.

WHAT IS CONSTIPATION?

Here's a definition of constipation from Wiktionary: A state of the bowels in which the evacuations are infrequent and difficult to pass, or the colon becomes filled with hardened faeces. Another definition is pooping less than three times a week.

HOW DOES THE BODY GET CONSTIPATED?

Food waste moves too slowly through the body and stays too long in the colon. The colon then absorbs water from the stool, leaving it dry and hard; as a result, more stool accumulates, and the rectum muscles have difficulty pushing it out of the body.

COMMON CAUSES OF CONSTIPATION

Idiopathic or functional (cause unknown); lack of fibre in the diet; lack of water (dehydration); a side effect of medication (especially Opioids); a symptom of other health problems such as a spinal injury or pelvic floor dysfunction; hormone changes in pregnancy; an imbalance of good and bad gut bacteria; trauma; stress and anxiety; *laxative abuse; *withholding or resisting the *urge to poop.*

* Both can cause a weakening in peristalsis known as a motility disorder and result in a lazy/sluggish bowel, also known as slow transit constipation (STC).

COMMON SYMPTOMS OF CONSTIPATION

Infrequent bowel movements; stools are hard, dry, and difficult to pass; straining to have a bowel movement; feeling everything hasn't been expelled; pain, cramps, or bloating in the abdomen; feeling sluggish or lethargic; loss of appetite; headaches; nausea; unable to sleep; hemorrhoids and anal fissures.

PERISTALSIS

o Peristalsis is a wave-like muscle contraction in the walls of the colon which moves food along the digestive tract.

o Sometimes, peristalsis doesn't work correctly in the colon and causes a motility disorder. Suppose it goes too slowly and results in constipation. In that case, it's known as slow transit constipation (STC) or a lazy/sluggish bowel. If it goes too quickly, the result is diarrhoea.

o IBS sufferers can have both constipation and diarrhoea.

o If you conduct a web search on how to quicken peristalsis, the results may show a *to-do* list. It may include eating more fibre, drinking more water, exercising thirty minutes daily, abstaining from meat, eating yogurt, and taking probiotics. Doing all of this may improve transit time in some people but may have a negligible effect on others; it's dependent on the underlying cause of constipation.

o High-fibre food triggers peristaltic movement by adding bulk that expands the abdominal walls. However, it can have the opposite effect and slow down peristalsis in some people.

o Fibre acts like a sponge, absorbing water, so if you increase your fibre, ensure you increase your water, or you may become dehydrated and more constipated.

BOWEL TRANSIT TIME

Bowel transit time is how long it takes for food to travel from the mouth to your digestive tract, then into the colon, and be excreted as stool. A good transit time is twelve to forty-eight hours. Longer than this would be a *slow transit time* indicating constipation. An effortless way to evaluate transit time at home is to eat a cup of cooked corn kernels or beets on their own and an hour apart from other food. Wait for the kernels to show up in a bowel movement or for the bowel movement to be purple from the beets. Take a note of the time food is eaten and the time of the bowel movement; the time in between is the transit time.

TITBIT 1: BIOFEEDBACK THERAPY

Biofeedback Therapy is performed in a clinic or hospital. It can help train people to change the behavior of the muscles in their pelvic floor and anal sphincter and enable them to defecate more easily. The therapy may involve an anal probe, rectal balloons, and a visual monitor for the patient to view the muscles working and not working. Studies have shown it has a high success rate in improving constipation in many people. Search the Web for more information on Biofeedback Therapy and have a look at videos on YouTube about Biofeedback and Electrical Stimulation for Constipation.

MY STORY: CONSTIPATION

As a child, I grew up in a house in Scotland with eleven people: my mum, dad, five brothers, and three sisters. I didn't have a problem living with ten people. Still, I had a problem with only one bathroom in the house, as whenever I had *the urge to poop*, someone else in the family was using it. In addition, I was an introverted child in an extroverted family and didn't fight for my place in the queue.

From four years of age, I had frequent upset tummies. Finally at seven years, I was rushed to the hospital for an operation to remove a suspected burst appendix. However, after the procedure, the surgeon said the cause of the stomach pain was constipation and not an infected appendix. So, every Sunday after church, my mum gave me a large tablespoon of a stimulant laxative, which meant I had a clear-out on Monday. She also fed me lots of fruit, and homemade soups full of vegetables and legumes, establishing a lifelong healthy eating habit for which I'm grateful. The laxatives and the fruits and vegetables helped me poop two or sometimes three times a week, but it was always with straining.

I have no recollection of pooping regularly in childhood. Then at school and later in the workplace, I was so embarrassed at how long I spent in the bathroom that I would *hold it in* and wait till I was home. I had no idea this was creating a problem in my intestines and would worsen my constipation in the long term.

In my mid-twenties, I had two children and, during the pregnancies, suffered severe constipation. I was prescribed laxatives which gave temporary relief, but I knew it wasn't a long-term solution. In my thirties, I read many books on constipation, looking for the root cause and what I could do about it. I learned about *withholding* or *resisting the urge to poop,* which can begin early in life when a child is embarrassed to use public bathrooms or doesn't like the *smelly* school bathrooms. I had a lightbulb moment as I read this and realised that when I was a child and had the *urge to poop*, and someone was using the family bathroom, I would *withhold.* Then at school, because I took so long in the bathroom, I withheld again till I was home to avoid embarrassment.

With more reading, I learned that when we eat, the muscles in the walls of our gut contract and relax. As a result, the food is moved forward in a wavelength motion known as peristalsis, which gives us the *urge to poop.* I resisted this urge by *withholding*, and through time those muscles weakened, resulting in slow transit constipation. Fast forward to March 2019, when I lost the *urge to poop.* I am certain it was caused by eating a low-carb diet for a year which you'll read about in Chapter 7, My Story. The scary thing about it was that nothing I'd done in the past to manage my constipation helped me with this new difficulty of having no *urge to poop.*

I was four years old when constipation started, and at the time of writing this (2022), I'm now sixty-nine. That's sixty-five years! It's incredible that the world can send a man to the moon but can't come up with a cure for constipation.

TITBIT 2: THE SQUATTY POTTY

One way to speed up transit time is using a Squatty Potty, a toilet stool that curves around the toilet's base. Placing your feet far apart on the surface raises the knees above the hips and puts the body into a squat; the rectum is then in the ideal position to poop. A scientific study showed that seventy percent of people who used a squatty potty had faster poops. Bobby Edwards from Utah invented it with his mum Judy. She had constipation and used a footstool in the bathroom to place her feet on but asked her son if he could design and make something better. So, he developed and manufactured the squatty potty and began selling it in 2011 from his garage. The sales were steady until 2015, when an online ad went viral, clocking up 100 million views, and sales took off. You can view the ad on YouTube with the bizarre title, "This Unicorn Changed the Way I Poop."

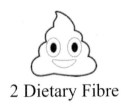

2 Dietary Fibre

FACT FILE: DIETARY FIBRE

A lack of dietary fibre can be a significant cause of constipation. Yet, fibre can worsen constipation in some people or cause digestive distress such as bloating and excessive gas.

WHAT IS DIETARY FIBRE?
o Dietary fibre is a complex carbohydrate, known as roughage or bulk.
o It's only found in plants and not in animal products.
o The human body lacks the digestive enzymes to break down fibre, so it simply passes through the digestive system and arrives in the colon intact.
o As the body doesn't digest fibre, it doesn't hold any calories.

WHAT FOODS HAVE DIETARY FIBRE?
o All plant foods have dietary fibre: fruits, vegetables, legumes (beans, peas, lentils, chickpeas), nuts, seeds, and wholegrains.
o Wholegrains are the seeds of cereal plants that have not been processed and contain all three parts of the grain: the bran, the endosperm, and the germ. Examples are barley, brown rice, buckwheat, bulgur (cracked wheat), millet, rye, maize, oatmeal, corn. In addition,

wholemeal bread, and wholewheat pasta are made from wholegrains.

o Wholegrains such as bread and rice are refined by removing the bran and the germ to make them 'white', leaving them devoid of fibre and many nutrients. The US and UK governments passed mandates stating that manufacturers must add nutrients to refined grains to replace what was lost in the refining process, hence the term 'fortified with' on the packaging of bread and cereals. Still, nutritionists say these nutrients are only a 'token' compared to the nutrients lost. Unfortunately, the government has not been concerned about manufacturers removing the bran (fibre).

HOW MUCH FIBRE SHOULD WE EAT?
Here are a few statistics from the Web.

o The UK and US governments recommend adults have 30g of fibre a day. Yet the average adult fibre intake is only 14g to 18g daily.

o According to age group, the recommended fibre intake for children is 2-5 years 15g per day; 5-11 years 20g per day; 11-16 years 25g per day.

o Water must be increased when fibre is increased, or stools may be hard and dry.

WILL THIRTY GRAMS OF FIBRE HELP ME POOP?

o The government recommendation of 30g of fibre a day isn't to help us poop (although it may do that) but to have a healthy, balanced diet. Too often, doctors quote this statistic to their constipated patients as the cure for constipation. Still, it's more a cure for an unhealthy diet.

o   Studies have shown the following benefits from eating a high-fibre, plant food diet: lower cholesterol levels, reduced blood pressure, reduced inflammation, more controlled blood sugar level, and lowered risk of cardiovascular disease and all cancers. Plant foods are full of the nutrients we need for a healthy body, although animal products also have many nutrients our bodies need except for fibre.

o   Some people eat a diet high in processed food and low in plant food. As a result, their fibre intake is less than the average of 14g to 18g a day, yet they don't have constipation. Eating less processed food and more plant food full of nutrients would benefit their health, and this is what the government hopes to achieve. Eating more plant food will increase their dietary fibre, but they may already be pooping without it.

SO HOW MUCH FIBRE SHOULD I EAT?

o   Our bodies are all different, so it's essential to work out for ourselves how much fibre in our diet will help us poop without causing digestive distress. We can do this by tracking our food, noting the amount of fibre we eat, and whether it's promoted a bowel movement. Also, we must consider if other compounds in our food such as gluten or specific foods such as beans are the culprits in our digestive distress. Fibre isn't always the bad guy!

HOW DOES FIBRE RELIEVE CONSTIPATION?

Fibre has two main components: soluble fibre and insoluble fibre (it does have others).

o   Soluble fibre absorbs water in the colon. It acts like a sponge, draws water into the stool, and becomes a gel-like substance in the gut, making it softer and easier to move through the digestive system. Colon bacteria ferment soluble fibre, and some of these bacteria create gas. Foods high in soluble fibre are oatmeal, barley, peas, beans, lentils, nuts, seeds, avocado, and some fruits and vegetables, including apples, oranges, berries, carrots, and sweet potatoes.

o Insoluble fibre does not absorb water in the colon. Instead, it is simply bulk that adds volume to the waste and gets it moving, pushing it through the digestive system. Studies have shown that insoluble fibre increases the dry mass of stools, but doesn't increase the stool's water content, and can therefore lead to constipation in some people. In addition, colon bacteria do not ferment insoluble fibre, so it doesn't cause as much gas as soluble fibre. Foods high in insoluble fibre are wholemeal bread and wholewheat pasta, brown rice, skins of apples and pears, most vegetables, and seeds.

SUMMARY
It's the job of the soluble fibre to make everything soft and easy to move, whereas it's the job of the insoluble fibre to push everything through. However, most plant foods have a mix of fibre for example apples are high in soluble fibre in the flesh and have some insoluble fibre in the skin.

FIBRE SUPPLEMENTS
o Fibre supplements are an easy and harmless way to increase fibre intake. They work by soaking up water in the gut, making the stool softer and easier to pass.

o It's recommended that a minimum of 250 ml of water be drunk with a fibre supplement and to drink plenty of water throughout the day.

o Start with a low dose and build up slowly to avoid digestive distress. If you suffer from intestinal diseases or are on medication, please speak with your doctor before taking them.

o Read the directions on your fibre supplement packet to check when to take it. In general, you should take them following your meal.

o Fibre supplements pass through the digestive system quickly, so don't take medication or nutritional supplements simultaneously. They may be carried to the colon and excreted before the body can absorb them.

POPULAR FIBRE SUPPLEMENTS

o Psyllium is a popular fibre supplement also known as Ispaghula. It's a fibre from the husks in seeds taken from the Plantago Ovata plant and contains 70% soluble fibre. However, many people find it unpleasant to drink, so an option is to take psyllium-based fibre supplements that have added flavouring and dissolve well in water. Examples of these are Metamucil, Fybogel, and Konsyl.

SUPPLEMENTS OTHER THAN PSYLLIUM

o BENEFIBRE: the main ingredient is wheat dextrin, a natural soluble fibre. Although wheat contains gluten, the wheat in Benefibre is so low that the manufacturer markets it as gluten-free. However, if you have gluten intolerance, it's best avoided.

o FIBRECON: this is made from a synthetic ingredient, calcium polycarbophil. The manufacturers say that it does not ferment in the colon like other fibre supplements and so does not cause excess gas. Also, many IBS sufferers find it beneficial in relieving their symptoms. It comes in tablet form but is not available in powder form.

o CITRUCEL: this is made from a synthetic form of cellulose, the primary substance found in plant cell walls. It's insoluble fibre, so it won't cause as much excess gas as supplements with soluble fibre.

o FIBRE GUMMIES: these come in a chewable tablet but are low in fibre, meaning you would have to eat a lot of gummies daily for adequate fibre; however, you don't need to mix them with water, so they are more convenient.

BUTYRATE

o Fibre does more than soften stools and move them along when it comes to constipation. The human body cannot digest fibre, so it reaches the colon unchanged. Once in the colon, it's digested by the good bacteria, which produces Butyrate, a short-chain fatty acid.

o Butyrate provides impressive benefits to the colon: an increase in stool transit time; a decrease in IBS symptoms; it's the fuel good bacteria use to multiply; it's the primary fuel source for Colonocytes, the cells that line the colon; it makes the colon more acidic and suppresses the growth of bad bacteria.

o Some food is high in Butyrate, such as butter, ghee, milk, and cheese; however, Butyrate is absorbed in the small intestine and doesn't reach the colon. Therefore, the best way to increase Butyrate production is to eat food high in soluble fibre: oatmeal, barley, peas, beans, lentils, nuts, seeds, avocado, and certain fruits and vegetables - apples, oranges, berries, carrots, and sweet potatoes.

o Conduct a Web search on Butyrate, and you'll be amazed at its many health benefits for the gut and our overall health. Butyrate supplements are also available.

IS IT POSSIBLE TO POOP WITHOUT FIBRE?

It may sound surprising, but people who follow a carnivore diet (meat only) manage to poop with zero fibre in their diet, although it isn't very often. You can read this in the Fact File in Chapter 7, *Low-Carb Constipation*.

TITBIT 3: ADDING FIBRE TO FOOD

In the 1970s, a British military surgeon, Doctor Dennis Burkitt, studied the health of rural Africans who ate up to 50g of fibre daily. He announced they had almost no colon cancer, diabetes, constipation, or IBS. He concluded this was because of their high-fibre diet, which came from starchy vegetables and one type of coarse grain. The Western media and food manufacturers then promoted an idea. Suppose everyone increased their fibre by adding wheat bran to their food or eating food that contained wheat bran, such as breakfast cereals and bread. In that case, they could be as healthy as the Africans. Unfortunately, they omitted to stress that Africans didn't add wheat bran to their food but ate a whole food diet. As a result, some people who added wheat bran to their food found it worsened their constipation.

MY STORY: DIETARY FIBRE

Constipation was a significant problem by the time I was thirty; I pooped once or twice a week and strained to pass incredibly hard stool. That was when I took laxatives which worked erratically. I was concerned about their long-term use and if they would harm my body. However, if I didn't take them, I worried about all the stool stuck in my colon and the painful hemorrhoids caused by straining. Eventually, I stopped taking laxatives and have recently read many posts on Facebook groups where members write that, in time, laxatives became ineffective in helping them poop. In addition, they caused irreversible damage to the colon in some people.

I noticed that I pooped more frequently if I ate high-fibre food. So, the bulk of my diet became vegetables, fruit, legumes (beans, peas, lentils, chickpeas), wholegrains such as oats, barley, wholemeal bread and wholewheat pasta. It was challenging to follow a vegetarian diet because I cooked for my family, so I settled on less meat with more vegetables for my evening meal. However, I needed discipline to eat high-fibre food and resist processed food. When I was sick, emotionally upset, on holiday, or celebrating, I lost that discipline and went days without pooping – I'm only human!

At this point, I resorted to a water enema rather than a laxative to clear my colon and returned to eating lots of high-fibre food. During this time, I began tracking my food to ensure I was eating enough fibre and drinking adequate water to manage constipation. Until I was sixty-five, this regime worked for me, and I could poop two or sometimes three times a week, depending on how much water and fibre I consumed.

Fast forward to March 2018, when I ate a low-carb diet for health reasons. Eating adequate fibre on a low-carb diet isn't easy, so I began taking two fibre supplements each day. I had one after breakfast and one after dinner, which was 7g daily. So along with the 23g of fibre I ate in my food, I ate 30g daily. However, low-carb vegetables have very little soluble fibre, so stool was often hard and difficult to pass. By March 2019, I was chronically constipated, and lost the *urge to poop*. I resorted to water enemas to have a bowel movement but was concerned that the enemas were ineffective some days. In the end, I decided to come off the low-carb diet and return to a diet high in soluble fibre. However, gas became so bad that I was nervous about leaving the house, and I still couldn't poop without a water enema. The only benefit was that the water enemas worked well when I ate high-fibre food.

I used a notebook to track my food to determine which food was causing the gas. The worst culprits were legumes: beans, peas, and lentils, which I ate in my homemade soups, and oats which I had most mornings for breakfast. However, I was concerned it would be challenging to eat enough fibre if I cut out the food causing gas. For example, a bowl of porridge was 6g of fibre, and a bowl of my homemade soup was between 6g-10g of fibre. All I could do was avoid eating legumes and oats before being in the company of other people. I also discovered smoothies at this time, and if I couldn't have homemade soup or oats because I would be with other people, I had smoothies that are easy to digest, high in fibre, and cause much less gas.

I read many articles on the web about gut health and learned about the gut microbiome and the importance of increasing the good bacteria in my gut. I experimented with fermented food, which has zero or little fibre but is full of good bacteria. I make Kefir all year and Sauerkraut only in the summer as I find it cold and unappealing in the winter. Water and coffee enemas became a big part of my regime, which I write about in Chapter 6.

There was one improvement. Homemade soups and smoothies gave less *bricklike* stool with water enemas. However, there was still no *urge to poop*, and I depended on enemas to clear my colon. Despite my efforts, I decided that there wasn't much improvement, and I needed something more. The something more was a Gut Test by Stool Analysis which you'll read about in Chapter 8.

TITBIT 4: FIBRE SUPPLEMENTS
Proctologist and Colorectal Surgeon Dr. David Rosenfield calls himself the number one butt doctor on the number two business in America. He recommends one teaspoon of psyllium a day in a glass of water to help constipation. He was a frequent guest on the Emmy award-winning program 'The Doctors" and has a YouTube channel with some of the videos from the program. (Proctologists are surgeons who deal with conditions in the anus and rectum, such as hemorrhoids, anal fissures, and abscesses).

3 Water

FACT FILE: WATER

Dehydration can be one of the significant causes of constipation. However, even if a large volume of water is drunk, constipation can still be a problem as many other factors are involved.

HOW DEHYDRATION AFFECTS STOOL
o If there isn't enough water in your body, the colon will soak up water from the food waste to maintain the body's hydration.
o Without adequate water, the stool formed will be dry, hard, and difficult to pass.
o If the body is hydrated, urine will range in colour from clear, pale yellow to gold and have no odour. If the body is dehydrated, urine will have a much deeper gold colour and a strong odour. However, a doctor should check any urine colour changes.

HOW MUCH WATER TO DRINK?
o Many factors affect how much water the body needs: the temperature of the weather, body weight, exercise, and your diet – up to twenty percent of your water intake comes from your diet.
o In 1945, the US Food and Nutrition Board recommended one millilitre for every calorie eaten. So, on a 2000-calorie diet for women, this would be two

litres, and on a 2500-calorie diet for men, this would be two and a half litres. Years later, they recommended six to eight glasses of water a day.

- Water can also be drunk in soups, herbal teas, and diluting squash or cordial. Cold water dilutes digestive enzymes and juices, whereas warm or hot water is gentler on the digestive system.
- Hot water with lemon juice works on the digestive system and gets things moving.
- Apple Cider Vinegar (ACV) makes the water more effective for digestion. ACV is made from the fermented juice of apples and contains significant amounts of pectin, a water-soluble fibre. Pectin normalizes the acid levels in the stomach and aids digestion which is said to help promote bowel movements. However, you must dilute ACV in water, or it weakens tooth enamel, leading to tooth decay.
- If you don't feel like drinking water, try going a few hours without food, and you'll become aware of your natural thirst; constant snacking masks our thirst.
- On Facebook support groups for constipation, some people post that when they drink three litres of water each day, they don't experience constipation. WARNING: studies show that drinking over three litres of water in a brief period can trigger a life-threatening condition. It's known as Hyponatremia, where the sodium content in your blood becomes diluted.

SPARKLING WATER
- Sparkling water (carbonated water) is water manufacturers inject with carbon dioxide gas under pressure.

o A study was conducted on twenty-one constipated people for fifteen days; they gave ten people tap water to drink and gave the rest sparkling water. The average bowel movement frequency in the group that drank sparkling water increased significantly. However, another study has shown that sparkling water may cause a flare-up of IBS.

o There's lots of information about studies on sparkling water on the Web. Conduct a Web search to learn more about the pros and cons of drinking sparkling water before trying it.

DIURETICS

o Diuretics are substances that increase the production and excretion of urine from the body through the kidneys. The body's then left with less water; the colon draws water from the waste, and the stools formed are hard and dry.

o Forced diuretics, known as water pills, stimulate the kidneys and form urine, making urination more frequent.

o Caffeine is a diuretic, so drinks containing caffeine - coffee, tea, cocoa, cacao, and cola can dehydrate the body. Energy drinks such as Red Bull have twice the caffeine as coffee.

o Alcohol is a diuretic, although it doesn't contain caffeine.

o Plants and herbs may contain caffeine, so always check the nutritional information on herbal teas.

o Cola has high acidity levels, and the body must use twice as much water as the *can* to deal with it.

- Some people find that an early morning caffeinated coffee triggers a bowel movement. Adding a tablespoon of MCT oil (medium-chain triglyceride) can be even more effective. Or add butter to make a Bulletproof Coffee (created by Dave Asprey). Others find drinking caffeinated green tea after a meal can loosen the bowels. However, caffeinated green tea and coffee can also constipate.

TANNINS

- Tannins (tannic acid), are naturally occurring plant compounds in some food and drink. Some of the richest sources of tannins are tea, coffee, wine, and chocolate.
- It's said that tannins provide antioxidant and anti-inflammatory benefits to our bodies. However, when it comes to constipation, they can disrupt the fluid balance in our guts, binding the stool and holding back the bowel movement.
- Black tea is much higher in tannins than green tea, and coffee has half the quantity of tannins as black tea.
- The number of tannins in tea and coffee depends on how it's produced and how long it's steeped.
- It would be difficult to tell if tannins in tea and coffee exacerbate your constipation. The best solution may be fasting from them for a period to see if it makes any difference. Another solution may be to avoid overconsumption.

SOME SIMPLE GUIDELINES TO FOLLOW

- Follow every diuretic drink with a cup of water.

- Be intentional. If you're based at home, fill a jug with the water you intend to drink each day, or if you're mobile, carry bottled water.
- Track your water to determine how much water you need to avoid *bricklike* stools.
- If you're following a low-carb diet, it's suggested to drink a minimum of two and a half litres of water each day.
- Consider cutting out drinks like cola completely.

TITBIT 5: SIPPING OR GULPING?
Research has shown that urine excretion is six times lower when water is regularly sipped instead of gulping down more significant amounts. As a result, there are fewer trips to the bathroom, and the body retains more water and stays hydrated. Therefore, only gulp water when your muscles need to be quickly hydrated, for example, by athletes training or competing.

MY STORY: WATER

I've always been a Tea Jenny. I drank copious cups of tea every day, unconcerned about it as I'd read that you could include tea in your water intake. Then a few years ago, I read on the Web that tea, coffee, and cola are diuretics (because of the caffeine) and flush fluids out of the body, resulting in constipation.

Learning this was a eureka moment for me as I'd been drinking lots of caffeinated green tea for its health benefits throughout the day. However, an online article referred to it as *green tea constipation,* so I switched to decaffeinated green tea, and my stools became less *bricklike.* Another tea I like is Redbush tea or Rooibos, made from a South African herb, which I think is the only herbal tea that comes close to the taste of *real* tea. If you're concerned about tannins in tea, then Rooibos tea is an excellent choice as it's low in tannins. However, I like the buzz I get from a cup of caffeinated tea, so I allow myself one weak tea in the morning and one when I eat out.

HERE'S HOW I DRINK WATER

o I tracked my daily water intake and discovered the quantity that worked for me was a minimum of one and a half litres a day. If I had less than this, it was back to *bricklike* stools. I aim for two litres a day, but I don't consistently achieve this.

o I start drinking water as soon as I'm awake and aim for one litre in the morning. If I don't do this, it's challenging to reach my daily quota. Also, I don't drink in the evening to avoid trips to the bathroom during the night.

o   I drink room temperature or hot water as it feels gentler on my insides than chilled water.

o   Many health experts say not to drink liquid with a meal as it's not good for digestion. However, I ignore this and have a glass of diluted squash or cordial with each meal. It's a simple way to ensure I'm drinking enough water.

o   I've always consumed hot water with lemon juice in the mornings, and I added Apple Cider Vinegar for a time. My recipe was ½ tablespoon lemon juice and ½ tablespoon ACV in 250ml water. However, after a while, I realized I wasn't drinking as much because I wasn't fond of the taste of ACV in the water, so I reverted to hot water and lemon juice.

o   Most days, I drink one litre of plain water, and the rest is in decaf tea, soups, and diluting drinks such as squash or cordial.

TITBIT 6: A VIBRATING CAPSULE TO HELP YOU POOP

You may think a vibrating capsule that helps you poop is a joke. Still, it may be a serious answer to constipation caused by slow peristalsis. An Israeli medical technology company called Vibrant has manufactured a tiny capsule programmed to vibrate twelve hours after it is swallowed and reaches the colon. The capsule (no bigger than a vitamin pill) is first put into a small pod to be activated. Twelve hours after it's swallowed, vibrations from the capsule induce peristalsis in the colon, and the person spontaneously poops. Ninety percent of people taking the pill doubled the number of their bowel movements.

However, Vibrant is still evaluating the capsules' long-term effects on peristalsis. In 2021 it was in trials with the US Federal Drug Administration. The company is currently working with investors to bring it to market, although they haven't said what it would cost. Here's their website address if you want to check it out: www.vibrantgastro.com

4 Nutritional Supplements

FACT FILE: NUTRITIONAL SUPPLEMENTS

WARNING: if you suffer from any medical conditions or are on medication, consult your doctor before taking supplements.

TESTING FOR VITAMINS AND MINERALS

You can purchase a home finger-prick blood testing kit for vitamin and mineral levels online. You can have your blood tested for Magnesium, Vitamin D, and Vitamin B12, which are said to help with constipation. I use the words *are said* as although research has shown that these supplements help with constipation, some people who've taken them haven't experienced any change in bowel movements. Our bodies are all different, and what works for one person may not work for another; therefore, we must decide for ourselves what to take.

NOTE: for a Vitamin C check, you must have your blood tested within one hour of being taken, so you would have it tested at a walk-in clinic.

MAGNESIUM

Magnesium is a mineral that relaxes the muscles in the intestines and draws water into the colon, which softens stool and makes it easier to pass. However, it's said that most of the Western population is deficient in Magnesium.

34

Studies have shown that Magnesium Citrate is the most effective Magnesium supplement for constipation. Other supplements, such as Magnesium Oxide, were not shown to be as effective. The recommended daily dose for constipation is 400 mg for men and 320 mg for women.

Here's a list of food high in Magnesium, starting with those with the highest levels: dark chocolate, pumpkin seeds, black beans, oatmeal, cashew nuts, avocado, baked potato with skin, flaxseeds and chia seeds, bananas, oily fish such as salmon or mackerel, and green leafy vegetables such as kale and spinach.

WARNING: people with heart disease, kidney disease, intestinal blockage or appendicitis, diarrhoea, and pregnant or nursing women should not take Magnesium without consulting their doctor.

VITAMIN C
Vitamin C speeds up the digestive process and enables food to pass quickly through the intestines, preventing stool build-up and increasing the frequency of bowel movements. The recommended dose for constipation is two 1000 mg tablets daily, one in the morning and one in the evening.

Here's a list of food high in Vitamin C, starting with those with the highest level: bell peppers, guava, citrus fruits, kiwi, broccoli, strawberries, leafy greens, cauliflower, and tomatoes.

VITAMIN B12

A deficiency of Vitamin B-12 can be a primary cause of constipation and irritable bowel syndrome. It can be taken in supplement form or given as an injection. It isn't present in plant food but is present in animal products. However, as we age, the body doesn't absorb it well from food, and studies have shown that most people over fifty years have a deficiency. The body also doesn't absorb it well from supplements, so the supplement level of B12 is much higher than the recommended daily allowance of 2.4 mcg for adults.

Here's a list of food high in Vitamin B12, starting with those with the highest level: beef liver, clams, oysters, mussels, tuna, beef, and dairy food such as milk, cheese, and eggs. For those who don't eat animal products, try Yeast Flakes, and breakfast cereals fortified with B12.

VITAMIN D

Studies have shown that a Vitamin D deficiency can be linked to chronic constipation caused by a motility disorder (slow transit).

However, studies show two instances when Vitamin D is the reason for constipation. First, taking an excess of Vitamin D can increase calcium levels in the blood, causing constipation. Second, if you take Vitamin D and your body lacks Magnesium, this can also cause constipation. So, a finger-prick blood test would reveal if there's an excess of Vitamin D in the body or if the body lacks Magnesium.

Vitamin D is the sunshine vitamin as the body makes it when the sun hits our skin. Unfortunately, like Magnesium, it's said that most of the population is deficient in this vitamin. The recommended daily allowance of Vitamin D starts at 400 IUs, but many take supplements up to 5,000 IUs.

Here's a list of food containing Vitamin D, starting with those with the highest levels: oily fish, red meat, liver, egg yolks, and fortified breakfast cereals, although it's challenging to get what the body needs from food alone as the levels of Vitamin D in food are low.

HERBS
Many people use herbs or herbal solutions for constipation, which may be something you'd like to try. Some examples are Cascara Sagrada, Slippery Elm, Aloe Vera, Fenugreek, and Dandelion. Also, always check the ingredients of herbal remedies for Senna, a known laxative. However, many also find that herbal products stop working after a time, known as habituation which means a diminishing response after prolonged, repeated use.

DIGESTIVE ENZYMES
Digestive enzymes are in our salivary glands and digestive tracts. They help break down large food molecules into smaller pieces so the body can easily digest them, and the cells absorb them. Taking digestive enzyme supplements helps the body digest food more efficiently, which can help constipation. In addition, different digestive enzymes help break down protein, fat, and carbs. Researching on the Web

would help you select the enzyme that suits your body's needs.

However, enzymes can be increased naturally by eating daily portions of raw fruits and vegetables or fermented food. Some foods high in natural digestive enzymes are pineapples, papayas, mangoes, kiwi fruit, bananas, avocados, ginger, sauerkraut, kimchi, and miso. Adding these foods to your diet may help promote digestion and better gut health. When food is eaten slowly and chewed thoroughly, the digestive enzymes have time to break down the food. Heat and cooking destroy enzymes. Highly processed food is deficient in enzymes and can cause undigested waste to ferment in the colon and attract bad bacteria.

NOTE: calcium and iron supplements can cause constipation.

TITBIT 7: INTERESTING FACTS ABOUT VITAMINS
VITAMIN B12: Beef liver is considered one of the most nutritious foods in the world. It's classified as nutrient-dense organ meat high in Vitamin B12 and other vital nutrients. A 100g portion contains an incredible 74mcg of Vitamin B12. The recommended daily allowance is 2.4mcg; however, the body stores any excess in the liver.
VITAMIN C: Over the centuries, multitudes of sailors died of scurvy when taking long sea trips until, in the 1600s, a military surgeon discovered that if the sailors ate citrus fruits, they didn't develop scurvy. However, it was two hundred years before the medical profession accepted this

and another hundred years before a chemist labelled the unknown substance that prevents scurvy as Vitamin C.

VITAMIN D: Research from the US has shown that of the people who died from Covid during the pandemic, seventy percent were deficient in Vitamin D. Because of Lockdown, many people stayed indoors; hence, their bodies could not produce Vitamin D from sunlight which led to Vitamin D deficiency.

MY STORY: NUTRITIONAL SUPPLEMENTS

After I stopped taking laxatives, I tried many vitamins, minerals, herbs, and enzymes. I spent considerable money on them, hoping to find a cure for my constipation. However, after several years without any change in constipation, I stopped everything except Vitamin C and Magnesium.

Over the years, I had used a Vitamin C flush to cleanse the bowel by taking a 1000 mg tablet every hour for six hours till I pooped. Based on this experience, I decided to take two 1000 mg tablets daily, one in the morning and one in the evening, the recommended dose to help with constipation.

At the beginning of my year of eating low-carb, I experienced painful muscle cramps in my legs during the night. I posted on a Facebook group asking for advice, and a member replied to supplement with Magnesium. I was taking a low dose of Magnesium, but once I increased it, the cramps stopped. I was then confident that supplementing with Magnesium was effective. Muscle cramps are common on low-carb diets, as they exclude many high-carb foods containing Magnesium. It's said that most of the population in the Western world is deficient in Magnesium which is possibly why the recommended daily dosage of 400 mg for men and 320 mg for women seems high.

I read on the Web that deficiencies in Vitamin B12 and Vitamin D can cause constipation. I then discovered that a simple finger-prick blood test could reveal whether the body was deficient in these vitamins. So, I purchased a Nutrition Test Kit online, which would test for Magnesium, Vitamin B12, Vitamin D, inflammation, cholesterol, and triglyceride levels. It cost £80 in 2022, and I also paid £30 to have blood taken for the test at a clinic as I can never get enough blood with a finger-prick.

My results came in a few days later. They revealed that Magnesium levels were normal, probably because I take a Magnesium supplement. However, I was deficient in Vitamin D and borderline low in Vitamin B12. So, I started taking a daily Vitamin D supplement of 4000 IU (International Units). After that, I considered having a Vitamin B12 injection costing £30 and lasting six months (the liver stores excess B12). However, I decided instead to eat liver once a fortnight, giving me a regular intake of B12.

I may retake the Nutrition Test in the future to check if things have changed for the better. The test also showed my HDL cholesterol was normal, but LDL cholesterol was too high, so I'm addressing this with my diet. I'd say the blood test was worthwhile, and I'm hopeful that, taking Vitamin D supplements along with eating liver for B12 will help with constipation in the long-term.

Regarding enzymes, I drink goat's milk Kefir all year and eat Sauerkraut in the summer. Both are high in enzymes.

TITBIT 8: VITAMIN C BOWEL FLUSH
To do the Bowel Flush, mix 1000 mg of buffered Vitamin C powder into some water and drink every hour. The body

absorbs powdered Vitamin C more quickly than 1000 mg tablets, but tablets also work for this flush. You'll have loose, watery poops when the body reaches saturation point, which may happen after five or six doses. Vitamin C is water-soluble, so the body doesn't store it. If you consume more than your body needs, the body excretes it in your urine. Conduct a web search for the many benefits of taking this flush. However, it would be best if you only did the flush occasionally as Vitamin C increases the number of Oxalates in the urine leading to kidney stones.

WARNING: people with kidney disease or kidney stones should not do this flush. If you suffer from chronic illnesses or are on medication, please check with your doctor first.

5 Exercise

FACT FILE: EXERCISE

On Facebook groups, some members post that exercise eases constipation. Still, others post they run three to five kilometres daily or work out at the gym five times a week, but it has zero effect on their constipation.

Suppose inactivity is causing or exacerbating your constipation, then exercise will help. However, it may not be effective if there are other underlying causes. Here are three reasons why exercise may help with constipation:
1. It speeds up the time it takes food to move through the digestive system resulting in pooping quicker.
2. It decreases the time stool is in the intestines meaning the body will absorb less water, avoiding hard stool.
3. Aerobic exercise can increase blood flow to the intestines helping peristalsis.

EXERCISING THE GUT
A better exercise for constipation may be an exercise targeting the gut. YouTube is an excellent source for videos on this topic. For example, search for *Intestine Exercises for Digestion;* these are breathing exercises based on Eastern Traditions. Or search for *Exercise for Constipation* demonstrated by Physiotherapists. Another exercise to search for is *Pelvic Floor Exercises for Constipation.*

Dysfunction of the pelvic floor muscles can cause constipation as it's difficult to poop if pelvic floor muscles are too tight. Exercise that targets the pelvic floor muscles can help this.

EXERCISING THE VAGUS NERVE

The vagus nerve stimulates peristalsis to push food along the intestinal tract, so it must be working effectively to help with slow transit constipation.

It's activated by manipulating our vocal cords which you can do in different ways. For example, you can gargle with water (twice a day for 30 seconds) or say 'OM' the yoga chant. Singing and laughing are also effective as they both manipulate the vocal cords. The vagus nerve is a fascinating part of our body, and you may like to do some research on the Web to find out more about it.

EXTERNAL MECHANICAL VIBRATION

I've read on the web about *external mechanical vibration devices* that increase the number of bowel movements in a week.

In the early 2000s, engineers in Israel developed a vibration device that attaches to the patient's abdomen with a belt surrounding the back. The device applied a kneading-like motion on the abdomen, which quickened peristalsis and increased the frequency of bowel movements. It was tested on thirty elderly patients from two nursing homes in Israel and Greece. The researchers asked the patients to use the device for twenty minutes each day for twelve weeks.

Their weekly bowel movements increased from 1.4 a week to 3.9 by the second week. The patients sustained this result for the twelve weeks of testing. Some of the patients continued with the device long-term. At six months and twelve months, the patients reported that they had sustained the increase in the frequency of bowel movements with no adverse physical effects. Unfortunately, the manufacturer discontinued it, which was disappointing as it was a reasonable price of £300. However, it may be manufactured again in the future.

Check out this website www.mowoot.com. The Mowoot is a desktop device with a belt that fits around the abdomen. It's advertised as a device that "generates an exo-peristaltic effect that moves the faeces." It's made in and delivered from Europe (Barcelona) and costs around £1200. However, Mowoot guarantees it will work and offers a 50-day trial; if there is no change in constipation, they promise a refund. In addition, the reviews of people who use the belt are positive.

If you search the Web for vibration machines to help with constipation, many results will come up. For example, companies advertise whole-body vibration machines costing over £2,200 to relieve constipation, reduce joint pain, and strengthen muscles and bones. They are available in some gyms and you could try one there.

A Tens machine (Transcutaneous Electrical Nerve Stimulation) is a small device with leads connected to electrodes or sticky pads that you place on your skin. It is battery-operated and sends tiny electrical impulses through the pads onto your body. The electrical impulses cause a tingling sensation and reduce the pain signals sent to the brain and spinal cords, resulting in the muscles relaxing and a decrease in pain.

When used to treat constipation, you place the electrodes on specific areas of the body surface known as the spinal ganglion that regulates peristalsis of the colon. The electrical impulses then stimulate peristalsis. Research shows that it is an effective way to stimulate peristalsis and increase the number of bowel movements in people with constipation.

Another option is a vibration belt such as Slendertone, used to tone the abdominal muscles.

TITBIT 9: OLIVE OIL AND FLAXSEED OIL
Olive Oil and Flaxseed Oil have been shown in studies to relieve constipation. The oil stimulates your digestive system and lubricates the stool as it passes through the colon. One tablespoon of oil on an empty stomach in the morning is recommended. If you don't like the taste, try adding a teaspoon of lemon juice. However, one tablespoon of oil is 120 calories, so consider that if you're concerned about your calorie intake.

MY STORY: EXERCISE

In my twenties and thirties, exercise was part of my life. I did a bit of jogging and worked out at the gym, but it did not affect my constipation. I exercise now by doing half an hour of walking outdoors and fifteen minutes of gentle resistance exercise several times a week. However, my reasons for doing this are more for general health than to help with constipation.

I had read information on the Web about vibration. So, as I thought it might help, I bought a hand-held, battery-operated massage gun. I used it to massage the area over my colon, thinking it might speed up peristalsis. Unfortunately, I have wear and tear on my hands, and I found it difficult to hold and move the gun over my abdomen for more than five minutes. So, after several weeks, I stopped using it; however, I think it might work for some people if they could sustain its use for fifteen minutes.

When I was reading about the Mowoot and vibration machines, I was interested but at the same time cynical about them working. Years of trying things that did not affect my constipation have made me like this! I don't want to spend a lot of money on something that may not be effective. It's good that the manufacturer gives a guarantee of a refund if it doesn't work but as it's delivered from Spain it could be complicated to return. I may look for a gym with a vibration machine and try that instead.

Another option is a vibration belt such as Slendertone, used to tone the abdominal muscles. I might consider asking for a vibration belt for Christmas or my birthday, and if it doesn't work for constipation, it may give me abs!

No doubt, like yourself, I get weary of everything I must do for constipation, such as eating high-fibre food, drinking water, and taking enemas. However, I think a vibrating belt or machine promoting pooping could be the answer, although it would depend on the cost. I'm hopeful of the vibrating pill that may be for sale soon, and I will be trying that.

TITBIT 10: COLOURED POOP

Poop can sometimes be a colour other than brown such as black, red, orange, green, or white/pale.

A baby's poop can be black the first few days after birth and yellow if breastfed. People with celiac disease can have yellow poop if they eat food with gluten.

Food such as licorice, dark green vegetables, and beets can change the colour of your poop, as can drinks with food colouring.

Medication or supplements can also change the colour of your poop. For example, Pepto Bismal taken for diarrhoea can cause pale-coloured poop, as can a barium meal taken before an x-ray. On the other hand, iron supplements and dehydration can cause black poop.

More serious reasons for a change of poop colour may be internal bleeding, digestive issues or your body isn't producing bile. Once you've determined you haven't ingested anything to change the colour of your poop, you should consult your doctor.

6 Enemas

FACT FILES: ENEMAS

If you've never taken an enema and are apprehensive about it, please wait until you're more comfortable with the idea. Join a Facebook group on enemas for help and support, read as much as you can on the Web, watch YouTube videos and discuss it with your doctor.

WHAT IS AN ENEMA?
The word enema comes from a Greek word meaning to inject. So, an enema is when fluid is injected into the rectum to clear out the bowel.

HISTORY OF ENEMAS
Water enemas aren't new. The first mention of enemas in medical literature was in a papyrus from Egypt written in 1600BC. It states that every Pharaoh had his *Guardian of the Anus* to perform his enemas. They used hollow reeds to direct water into the rectum. Moving forward to 500BC, Hippocrates and his followers in Greece also prescribed enemas as essential to good health. Then by the 17th century in Europe, Louis the 14th and his court are said to have taken frequent enemas, and enema jugs were a popular household item.

Medical professionals have used enemas for bowel cleansing before a medical procedure for many years.

Enemas have also been used consistently as home remedies, and in recent years, they've grown in popularity with people seeking alternative treatments to Western medicine.

WHY TAKE AN ENEMA FOR CONSTIPATION?
Every year in the UK, 56,000 people visit a hospital emergency department for constipation, and in the US, the number is 703,000. These numbers exclude those admitted to a hospital for treatment of constipation.

On Facebook Groups, people share how they checked into the emergency department of a hospital because of abdominal pain from fecal impaction. They usually haven't had a bowel movement for seven to fourteen days and write of how embarrassed and humiliated they were by the experience. When treating constipation at a hospital or doctor's surgery, a nurse or doctor administers a soap-suds enema and digitally removes the faeces, or the patient is given laxatives and sent home without treatment.

Taking an enema to clear the bowels instead of a laxative can give you time to focus on lifestyle changes without being anxious about a lack of bowel movements or the effect of laxatives on the body. People can fear taking enemas, yet on the Facebook group 'Coffee Enema Support,' many share they've been taking daily coffee enemas (for health) for 20, 30, and even 40 years and still have natural bowel movements. Enemas are often seen as a last resort to clear the bowel rather than seeing laxatives as a last resort.

Checking into an emergency department at a hospital could be avoided by taking a water enema on the third day without a bowel movement. However, leaving it for more than three days means the enema may be ineffective because hard faeces have impacted the colon. As a result, some people who try enemas say, "they don't work for me." Many take enemas when there hasn't been a bowel movement for several days. Others take them more frequently, even daily.

ENEMA EQUIPMENT
You can take an enema using either an enema bag or bucket.

o Bags are lightweight and more compact for travelling. You can easily hang them from something in the bathroom and see the liquid level through the plastic. However, if not cleaned thoroughly, coffee enemas can cause mould in the bag's seams.

o Buckets are more hygienic and easier to clean than bags. However, if it's a metal bucket, you can't see the liquid level going down, and as the tubing is 13mm up from the base, it must be tilted with your hand to be emptied.

TYPE OF WATER TO USE IN AN ENEMA
o If you take enemas frequently and long-term, it's best to use Distilled Water, either purchased in bottles or made in a home distiller. The distillers are electric and boil the water to capture the steam and then condense the steam back to water; distillation removes 99% of all contaminants.

o Many people use bottled Spring Water for their enemas. It's taken from under the ground and is considered pure; however, impurities such as heavy metals and nitrates can still be present.

o Reverse Osmosis Filters installed under the sink will not remove all toxins such as fluoride. Eleven percent of the population in the UK live in an area where the water is fluoridated. You can check online if the government fluoridates the drinking water in your area.

o Tap water contains contaminants and is not recommended for enemas. However, if you decide to use it, always boil it first.

HOW TO TAKE AN ENEMA

o First, close the valve on the tubing of the enema bag/bucket and fill with one litre of lukewarm water.

o Open the valve briefly to allow the water to flow to the tip of the nozzle and close it again. If you don't do this, the air will enter the rectum, and you'll pass gas all day.

o Hang the enema bag from the door handle, a towel rail, or the toilet paper holder. The bottom of the bag should be about 50cm above you to enable the water to flow easily. If it's higher than this, it can enter the colon too quickly, and the body will push it out. If you're using a bucket, place it on a stool or chair.

o For easy insertion, lubricate the nozzle with coconut oil.

o To take the enema, lie on the floor on your left side (rectum and anal canal are on the left side),

o Insert the nozzle gently into the anus, open the valve to release the water, and the water will flow into the colon. The water softens the impacted stool and stimulates a bowel movement; then, move to the toilet to defecate.

- Do not retain an enema for more than thirty minutes.
- One litre of water is recommended for enemas, although some articles on the Web recommend two litres of water. However, you may find that more water causes gurgling and churning in the colon after the enema. Try different quantities of water and decide what works best for you.

DIFFICULTIES TAKING ENEMAS

- If you suffer from hemorrhoids or fissures, you may experience pain when inserting the enema nozzle. If so, then have a look at the website of *Optimal Health Network*. They sell essential oils used in rectal suppositories with coconut oil as a carrier. Essential oils can support healing for colon-related ailments. In addition, the website has videos with clear instructions on how to make the suppositories.
- Suppose an enema doesn't stimulate a bowel movement. A tip is to lie on your back and massage the stomach area over the colon, especially the left side, where stool can be stuck and isn't moving into the rectum. Type *colon massage* into the search bar on YouTube for videos by Physiotherapists on colon massage.

DIFFERENT TYPES OF ENEMAS

SOAP-SUD ENEMA: this is the enema that a hospital or doctor's surgery may administer for constipation. The soap irritates the lining of the intestines much like a laxative and promotes a bowel movement. Like laxatives, it should only be for occasional use. Use a pure liquid soap such as Dr Bronner Castile Soap. You can buy it on Amazon but be aware that in large bottles of liquid economy soap, the soap is diluted. Start with one tablespoon of soap in one litre of warm water and gradually increase until you have the *urge to poop*. Some people find it stings slightly, especially if they have hemorrhoids or fissures, so start with one teaspoon and increase if you feel comfortable.

SALT-WATER ENEMA: adding salt to the enema water makes it more like body fluid and lets you retain it longer than a plain water enema. To make the enema solution, mix one to two tablespoons of Celtic or Himalayan salt with one litre of warm water. Salt-Water Enemas are not recommended for long-term use as they may disturb the microflora in the colon and lead to intestinal problems.

COFFEE ENEMA: these are primarily for detoxing the liver. The coffee remains in the colon, but phytonutrients from the coffee travel through the colon veins to the liver. They increase the production of glutathione (a powerful antioxidant that reduces cell damage) and help in releasing detoxifying bile. If taken over a long time, it's said that coffee enemas can tone the intestines, improve peristalsis, and cleanse the colon lining. However, there is no research to confirm this.

You make them by mixing one litre of water with three tablespoons of organic ground coffee. Next, boil the liquid for five minutes, then simmer gently with the lid on for fifteen minutes. Once it's cooled down, the solution is put through a strainer (filter) a few times to remove the coffee grounds. It's then taken as an enema lying on the right side (the liver is on the right side) and held for twelve to fifteen minutes; this is the recommended time to detox the liver. However, for the coffee to be retained in the bowel, you must take it with an empty colon, so one or two water enemas may have to be taken before taking the coffee enema to clear the colon.

WARNING: coffee enemas should only be retained for 15 minutes and taken a few hours apart, never back-to-back.

Coffee enemas also stimulate the lining of the intestines and trigger a bowel movement. To use them to clear the colon, make the enema solution as described above but lie on your left side (as in a water enema). Suppose the coffee enema works quickly but only partially clears the colon. In that case, you might try dividing it into two half litre enemas and take them back-to-back.

Join the *Coffee Enema Support Group* on Facebook, which has sixteen thousand members and files with all the necessary information to take coffee enemas. It's a friendly group, and they will answer any questions you may have on coffee enemas.

FLEET ENEMA: this is one of the most potent enemas. It's a saline (salt) laxative and draws water into the colon, which helps produce a bowel movement. It comes in a disposable plastic bottle with a lubricated tip. The solution is applied rectally by squeezing the bottle. It only takes two to five minutes to feel the strong urge to evacuate. However, doctors do not recommend them for the elderly or infirm.

COLONIC IRRIGATION: a Colon Therapist administers what's known as a *colonic*. It involves flushing waste material out of the colon using a large amount of water. Here's the procedure: the therapist explains what happens and takes a brief medical history; you're given a gown to wear and asked to remove your clothing from the waist down; you lie on a padded treatment table; the therapist inserts the tip of a long tube attached to the irrigation equipment into the rectum; the colon is gently flushed with repeated doses of warm water, which loosens waste and then filters it out through a closed tube system; the therapist can see the waste moving through and out of the tube but not the client; there is no odour; the only discomfort is slight cramping in the abdomen just before the waste is expelled.

A colonic thoroughly cleanses the whole colon and removes any old waste attached to the colon lining. The session lasts about forty-five minutes and costs £60 in 2021. Many people use colonics to clear the bowel of a blockage or impacted stool. However, as far as is known, it doesn't improve peristalsis or offer any benefits for long-term constipation.

PERISTEEN ANAL IRRIGATION SYSTEM: this is a transanal irrigation system for people who suffer from long-term chronic constipation. The person or caregiver uses the hand pump (part of the system) to flood the colon with water. It's used on alternate days and works quickly, cleansing much more of the colon than an enema. There's a video on YouTube – "Peristeen" by Doctor Anton Emmanuel, which explains how it works and has pictures of the equipment. The company that supplies it is *Coloplast*, although you must purchase it with a doctor's prescription. Here are their websites: www.coloplast.us and www.coloplast.co.uk.

CARE WITH ENEMAS

There is little scientific research on the adverse effects of taking enemas. What you can read on the Web is anecdotal; however, you must take care to avoid the following complications:

○ Burning the colon lining with hot water: the water should be around body temperature or lukewarm; use a bath thermometer to check the temperature of the water; the typical human body temperature range is 36.5–37.5C; many people find 40C comfortable.

○ Frequent use may cause an electrolyte imbalance: electrolytes in the blood are salts and minerals such as sodium, potassium, magnesium, and chloride. You can buy magnesium in tablet form; you can take potassium and sodium in Low Salt; chloride, and sodium in Himalayan or Celtic Salt. Take them with water, not on an empty stomach, as it may cause nausea. Conduct a Web search to determine how much of these electrolytes to take. If you have any health problems or take medication, please check with your doctor first; many people who take frequent enemas drink Coconut Water with potassium, sodium, and manganese.

○ Loss of good bacteria: if you use enemas frequently, take a probiotic supplement, or eat fermented food to replace the good bowel bacteria, you may lose with the enemas.

- Dehydration: on the days you take an enema, drink more water than usual as the enema may cause dehydration.
- Damaging the rectum: always gently insert the nozzle into the rectum and lubricate it with coconut oil for easy insertion; rubber catheters (latex) are soft, flexible, and comfortable and help avoid damaging the rectum with frequent use; it's particularly recommended for daily coffee enemas as it can be inserted 15cm to 20cm into the rectum and helps the phytonutrients in the coffee reach the liver; you can buy them online from Midwest Health and Nutrition Inc based in the US. They are not available in the UK.

NOTE: when using the red catheter for water enemas, don't insert it more than 8 cm to 10 cm, or you may weaken the peristaltic muscles further up the rectum with frequent use. However, once your bowel is empty, it's ok to insert the catheter 15 cm to 20 cm to get the full benefit of a detox coffee enema.

HOW TO CLEAN ENEMA EQUIPMENT

Clean the enema equipment with warm soapy water by letting the water run through the bag/bucket and the tubing. The tip can be taken off and washed separately; use a narrow bottle brush to clean it thoroughly. The enema equipment can also be left to soak in a bath. Leave the equipment to air dry by hanging from a hook for at least eight hours; this is important to prevent mould from forming in the tubing. For a thorough cleanse, pour three percent undiluted hydrogen peroxide into the bag/bucket. Once it reaches the tip, close the clamp. Leave the hydrogen peroxide in the tubing for a minimum of two and a half hours; it's safe to leave it overnight. Then, rinse the equipment thoroughly to remove any hydrogen peroxide residue.

WARNING: some people have forgotten the tubing is filled with Hydrogen Peroxide, topped it up with water, and then taken an enema. Hydrogen Peroxide can burn the intestinal lining, not seriously but enough to cause discomfort for several days. Therefore, ensure you rinse the bag and tubing thoroughly.

TITBIT 11: HOW TO MANUALLY CLEAR AN IMPACTION
This method will only work for impactions in the rectum or lower down in the colon. You can clear the stool yourself digitally using a lubricated, gloved finger. Also, women can insert a gloved finger into the vagina, pushing against the wall with the stool behind and moving it down. Search the Web for a Disimpactor device. It's like a long flexible arrow with the top part having fins. You insert it into the anus, and the head of the device enters the fecal impaction allowing you to have traction to remove the stool in fragmented pieces. You can follow this procedure with an enema to remove stool further up the colon.

MY STORY: ENEMAS

I began taking water enemas over thirty-five years ago when I stopped taking laxatives. I read a book on constipation by a doctor who wrote that taking water enemas was preferable to taking laxatives or straining to poop as both may harm the body. So, if I hadn't pooped for a few days because I'd been eating processed food and not drinking enough water, I took a water enema to clear my bowel instead of a laxative. It was like starting again, and I immediately got back on track with high-fibre food and water.

If I left it longer than a few days, the stool became *bricklike,* and the water enema was ineffective. When this happened, I took a soap-suds enema and did two or three enemas back-to-back till my bowel was clear. In the years before my colon shut down, the frequency of pooping would be anything from thirty-six to seventy-two hours. I want to stress that I did not take regular daily enemas; I only took an enema if I'd gone more than sixty hours without pooping which could be once every few weeks. However, when I lost the *urge to poop* after following a low-carb diet, I took water and coffee enemas daily for four months, then switched to alternate days because of the time involved.

It was awkward and uncomfortable lying on the bathroom floor when I began taking frequent enemas. Then, I read a Facebook post that suggested using pillows inside plastic bin liners, making it a much more comfortable experience.

Although I've read on the web that you can retain a water enema for thirty minutes, I only retain them for fifteen minutes. My experience is that if they're not effective in the first fifteen minutes, they won't be effective after that. So, if the enema doesn't work, I use a fresh warm enema solution with liquid soap.

I had a friend of eighty-four who fell and broke her hip and was admitted to the hospital for a hip replacement. She also suffered from chronic constipation and was unable to poop after her operation. The hospital gave her large doses of laxatives over two days till her bowels moved. Unfortunately, she didn't make it from the bed to the bathroom. She said the mess on the floor and the foul odour was horrendous, and she was so humiliated by the experience that she couldn't stop crying. I would hate to experience that, and I'm grateful I discovered enemas.

For over thirty-five years, enemas have helped me avoid straining to pass *bricklike* stool, which can lead to hemorrhoids and anal fissures. I suffered from painful hemorrhoids before taking enemas but not since then.

I watched a YouTube video, and someone mentioned that coffee enemas could restore good bowel tone and improve peristalsis. However, I didn't find any research that confirmed this, but it got my attention. So, after conducting a Web search, I began taking daily coffee enemas in July 2019. I read that they're for detoxing the liver (the largest organ in the body), improving health, stimulating the intestines, promoting bowel movements, and cleansing the colon. Initially, I didn't want to do coffee enemas as I was a bit nervous about putting *coffee up my butt*; it seemed a bit mad. However, the Facebook group *Coffee Enema Support* gave me the support and information I needed to get started.

So, what was my experience with coffee enemas? Once I saw the benefits of cleansing my colon and the feeling of well-being after the coffee enema (the effects of the caffeine), I decided to continue with them long-term. However, as the enema is retained for fifteen minutes to cleanse the liver of toxins, you must empty the bowel first. So, I had to take one or two water enemas before the coffee enema, which meant setting aside an hour in the morning to do this.

Around this time, I made three purchases. The first was a red rubber/latex catheter to replace the plastic nozzle on the enema tubing, a game-changer for comfort. The second was an electric water distiller to give me peace of mind that I wasn't filling my colon with contaminants from the water, before this, I used boiled tap water. My third purchase was a Squatty Potty which I found effective.

The main benefit of taking coffee enemas was that the unpleasant odour from my colon decreased in the first week. Over the months, some odd stuff appeared in the stool, dislodged from the colon wall. So, the cleansing side worked, although I didn't notice any difference in transit time or frequency of pooping. I recently read that coffee enemas can improve peristalsis if taken for two years; however, the article didn't quote any research to support this. After four months of daily coffee enemas, I switched to alternate days because of the time involved.

ENEMA BAG OR BUCKET?

For decades when I took an occasional enema, I used a plastic enema bag, easily purchased from pharmacies or on the Web and simple to use. You can hang them on the bathroom door handle or the toilet paper holder. They're easy to pack in a suitcase for holidays. Then, when I took coffee enemas, I switched to a metal bucket. I'd read that coffee can form mould in an enema bag's seams if not cleaned thoroughly. However, one drawback with the metal bucket is that you can't see the liquid reducing (you can see it in a plastic bag or transparent plastic bucket). Another drawback in using the bucket for coffee enemas is that it's difficult for the last bit of liquid to flow out because of the tubing position. The problem with this is that the phytonutrients in the coffee can settle at the bottom of the bucket. However, if you can reach the bucket, it can be tipped slightly, so the liquid enters the tube, although my attempts at this have sometimes resulted in tipping the coffee over myself.

COLONIC IRRIGATION

After taking coffee enemas daily for four months, I visited a Colon Therapist for colonic irrigation, which involves flushing waste material out of the colon using a large amount of water. I'd read that coffee enemas can dislodge old waste material on the colon walls, and colonics can remove this. After the colonic, the therapist told me that a hard piece of waste had come out, which she said may have caused a blockage in the future.

The colonic released a vast amount of waste, and for the first time in my life, I experienced an empty colon, and I felt ten-pounds lighter! The only discomfort was slight stomach cramps just before my body expelled the waste. Also, I felt physically tired and drained after it, but this passed after a good night's sleep.

From my experience and the experiences of others on Facebook groups, I'd say that a colonic clears the bowel and may remove blockages but doesn't do anything for constipation in the long term. I would have a colonic in the future if I thought I had a bowel blockage or a bowel impaction. Overall, I'd say the colonic was a good experience, and I recommend them for having a clear-out.

TITBIT 12: HISTORY OF COFFEE ENEMAS

Towards the end of World War One in Europe, there was a shortage of freshwater supplies, morphine, and other pain killers. The story goes that a nurse topped up an enema solution with the coffee available for surgeons to help them stay awake because of the limited water supply. As a result, the soldier who received the enema said his pain level had reduced. After the war, two German scientists investigated this. They found that caffeine entered the liver during the enema via the portal system and caused an increased bile flow, which released and evacuated accumulated poisons and toxins from the body. In the 1950's Dr. Max Gerson researched the work of these scientists and incorporated coffee enemas into his cancer therapy to clear the body of toxins.

7 Low Carb Constipation

FACT FILE: LOW-CARB CONSTIPATION

WHAT IS A LOW-CARB DIET?

- A low-carb diet limits the number of carbs consumed. The most popular low-carb diet is the Keto Diet, short for Ketogenic, restricting carbs to 20g daily. (Keto sounds Keeto).
- With only twenty percent of calories from carbs, the diet can be deficient in fibre, especially soluble fibre, unless carefully planned to include carbs with adequate fibre.

HOW CAN I GET ADEQUATE FIBRE ON A LOW-CARB DIET?

- Low-carb diets exclude most food typically eaten for fibre: root vegetables, fruits, whole-grains, legumes, brown rice, wholemeal bread and wholewheat pasta.
- However, some low-carb plant food can provide fibre: berries, rhubarb, avocado, chia seeds, flaxseeds and nuts, also vegetables grown above the ground such as broccoli, Brussel sprouts, and cauliflower. In addition, low-carb baking uses almond flour, coconut flour, and psyllium, all containing fibre.
- Taking a fibre supplement twice a day can help increase fibre intake.

o If constipation is an ongoing problem, you may have to increase your carb limit and include food with soluble fibre, such as apples.

THE EFFECT OF LOW-CARB ON CONSTIPATION?
According to Facebook groups, people's experience with constipation while eating low-carb can vary. For example, some who were already constipated said their constipation worsened, yet others said they started having regular bowel movements. In addition, people who'd never had trouble pooping became constipated after a brief time eating low-carb.

A ZERO FIBRE DIET BUT WITHOUT CONSTIPATION
Some low-carb eaters are carnivores (meat only) with zero fibre in their diet. Others who eat some carbs have less than 10g of fibre a day, yet they don't suffer from constipation. When following a *well-formulated keto diet* (WFKD), the body is always in ketosis. The liver then produces beta-hydroxybutyrate, which can replace some dietary fibre functions and the person can poop without constipation. If you'd like to know more about WFKD, check out this blog post: https://blog.virtahealth.com/fibre-colon-health-ketogenic-diet/ or search for *a well-formulated keto diet* on the web.

Here are lists of low-carb food with carb and fibre content. Always check the manufacturer's nutritional labels for the exact values on the packaging.

Vegetables with net carbs per 100g (3.5oz) followed by net fibre:
Asparagus 1.7g/2.1g; aubergine 2.9g/3g; bean sprouts 4g/2g; bok choy 3g/1g; broccoli 4g/2.6g; brussels sprouts 5g/3.8g; cabbage 3.3g/2.5g; cauliflower 3g/3g; celeriac 4.5g/1.8g; celery 1.3g/1.6g; cucumber 3.1g/0.5g; green beans 4.2g/2.7g; kale 5.2g/3.6g; lettuce 1.5g/1.3g; mushrooms 2.2g/1.0g; okra 4.2g/3.2g; olives 0.5g/3.3g; onions 7.6g/1.7g; parsley 3g/3.3g; peas sugar snap 5g/2.6g; pepper, red 3.9g/2.1g; pepper, green 3g/1.7g; pumpkins 6g/0.5g; radish 1.8g/1.6g; rutabaga 7g/2.3g; spinach 1.4g/2.2g; swede 6.3g/2.3g; swiss chard 2.1g/1.6g; tomatoes 2.7g/1.2g; turnip 4.6g/1.8g; zucchini 2.1g/1g.

Fruit with net carbs per 100g (3.5oz) followed by net fibre:
Avocado 1.8g/6.7g; blackberry 4.3g/5.3g, raspberry 5g/.5g; rhubarb 2.7g/1.8g; strawberry 5g/2g.

Nuts with net carbs per 100g (3.5oz) followed by net fibre:
Almond 6.9g/7.4g; brazil 4.2g/7.5g; coconut 6.3g/11.5g; hazelnut 7g/9.7g; macadamia 5.6g/8.6g; peanuts 7.6g/8.5; pecan 4.3g/9.6g; pine 9.4g/3.7g; walnut 7g/6.7g.

Nut products with net carbs per 100g (3.5oz) followed by net fibre:
Almond flour 6.9g/7.4g; coconut flour 6.3g/11.5g; unsweetened almond milk 0g/0.4g; almond butter 3g to 8g/ approx. 9g fibre; peanut butter 10g to 15g carbs/approx. 7g fibre.

Seeds with net carbs per 100g (3.5oz) followed by net fibre:

Chia seeds 11g/31g; flaxseeds 1.6g/27.3g; hemp 3.3g/27g; pumpkin 4.7g/6g; sesame 11.6g/12g; sunflower 18g/6g.

TITBIT 13: THE ELIXIR OF LIFE
Water is odourless, transparent, and tasteless, yet it's crucial for the body. The average human body is around sixty percent water; dehydration begins after only a few days without water. After that, the body experiences extreme thirst, fatigue, organ failure, and death between the third and seventh day. So, it's not surprising that it's referred to as the Elixir of Life. The keto diet causes a drastic decrease in carb intake. The problem with this is that water absorbs carbs. Without carbs to hold onto, the body excretes the water quickly, leading to dehydration. To combat this, a minimum of two and a half litres of water should be drunk daily when following a low-carb diet.

MY STORY: LOW-CARB CONSTIPATION

Many people eating low-carb have successfully lost excess weight and improved their health worldwide. I'm all for low-carb eating and in no way want to condemn it. What I've written here is simply my story of the effect low-carb eating had on my constipation.

From March 2018, for one year, I followed a low-carb Ketogenic Diet, Keto for short, with carbs limited to 20g a day. I have an autoimmune disease that causes swollen, painful joints. In only six weeks, the inflammation and the soreness lessened quite a bit. As well as this, I experienced a massive boost in energy, increased mental clarity, decreased cravings for sweet food, and a great night's sleep. A bonus was a seven-pound weight loss, so naturally, I was delighted!

When I began eating Keto, I was amazed to have regular soft poops; this was the only time I can remember this happening in my life. Sadly, after several weeks they stopped. There are two reasons why this may have occurred, but they are merely speculation.

First, the high fat in my diet, which was seventy percent of my total calories, may have caused the soft poops. Then my body may have adapted to the high fat and reverted to its constipated state. Second, the regular pooping may have stopped because I switched from what's known as *Strictly Keto* to *Easy Keto*. I started having artificial sweeteners and low-carb food with additives such as colours, flavour enhancers, emulsifiers, stabilisers, and preservatives. As I explained in the Fact File, a *well-formulated keto diet* (WFKD) keeps the body in a constant state of ketosis. The liver then produces beta-hydroxybutyrate, which replaces some dietary fibre functions. So, introducing artificial sweeteners and additives may have lowered my body's ketosis level. Then the liver stopped making beta-hydroxybutyrate, and regular pooping ceased.

So, with a return of constipation, I had to rise to the challenge of eating 30g of fibre a day while eating only 20g of carbs. I used a food tracker and included as many low-carb, high-fibre foods as possible to keep my fibre intake high. After breakfast and dinner, I took a fibre supplement, giving an additional 7g of fibre. This strategy worked for ten months apart from my usual bouts of constipation because I hadn't eaten enough fibre or drunk enough water. However, severe constipation kicked in towards the end of my year of eating Keto.

Pooping became less frequent; an unpleasant odour appeared on my breath and a more pungent odour from my colon when I pooped. Then, suddenly my bowels stopped working, and I lost the *urge to poop*. Finally, I resorted to daily water enemas to clear me out, but I had to have multiple enemas some days, which concerned me.

I loved eating low carb because of the energy and health improvements. Still, I decided my colon health was more important, and reluctantly one year after I started, I gave up low-carb eating. I returned to how I previously ate, all fruits and vegetables, legumes, wholemeal bread and wholewheat pasta, so there was an immediate increase in fibre, especially soluble fibre. The enemas were then effective, which relieved me, but I still had no *urge to poop.*

From reading on the web, I discovered that low-carb eating could cause the good bacteria in the colon to die off, and the bad bacteria then multiply and overpopulate the bowel. Then I read another online article about the role of the appendix in the body; remember, I had mine removed at age seven. I'd always read the appendix was a useless organ, but research now shows its role is to store good bacteria. If the colon becomes overpopulated with bad bacteria, the appendix releases its good bacteria to rebalance the colon. Discovering this information was another light bulb moment. I realized that my body couldn't address the imbalance in good and bad bacteria without an appendix, which was probably the cause of losing the *urge to poop.*

So, having learned this, my focus became repopulating the good bacteria in my colon through probiotics in food and supplements, which you'll read about in the following chapters.

TITBIT 14: ORIGINS OF THE KETO DIET
In America, in the early 1920's doctors discovered that when they put children who had Epilepsy on a fast, their seizures ceased. However, when they came off the fast, their seizures returned. Doctor Russell Wilder of the Mayo Clinic guessed that a diet could mimic fasting and designed the Classic Ketogenic diet. He placed children with Epilepsy on his diet, and after a short time, they moved into a state of ketosis. They burned fat instead of carbohydrates to produce energy. It was at this point that many of the

children's seizures ceased. Doctors successfully treated Epileptic children with the Ketogenic Diet for over 20 years until the medical community introduced anti-convulsant medications. Fast forward to 1972 when Doctor Robert Atkins published his book "The New Diet Revolution." He flew in the face of conventional dietary guidelines and drastically reduced the number of carbs in his Atkins Diet. As a result, many people lost weight and improved their health.

8 The Microbiome and Gut Tests

FACT FILE: THE MICROBIOME AND GUT TESTS

THE GUT MICROBIOME

o The gut microbiome is a community of around forty trillion microbes that live in the gut, more than any other area in the body. Scientists say the number of microbes equals the number of human cells in our body.

o Microbes are mainly bacteria with some viruses, protozoa, yeasts, and fungi.

o The gut or gastrointestinal tract is a passage from the mouth to the anus. It's where the body digests our food and then expels it as faeces when it reaches the anus.

o Most of the bacteria in the gut reside in the colon.

o The bacteria in the colon perform distinct functions: they help digest our food, protect against other disease-causing bacteria, produce essential vitamins, and help develop our immune system.

o Many gut specialists now believe the answer to chronic constipation and other gut issues is to develop a healthy gut microbiome.

GUT TEST BY STOOL ANALYSIS

o When it comes to constipation, it's essential to know what your gut microbiome consists of, and a gut test by stool analysis will reveal exactly that. In addition, the stool analysis results will give you the knowledge you need to address the specific issues in your colon that may be causing or worsening your constipation.

o To take a gut test, request a gut test kit from one of the many online gut health companies (or check with your doctor if you can have a free gut test). The kit will include the equipment you need for the stool sample and instructions on doing it. You then return the sample in a prepaid envelope, and within three to six weeks, you'll have your results.

o Depending on which test you buy, you may also receive recommendations on nutritional supplements and lifestyle changes for your specific gut issues.

TESTING FOR COMMON GUT ISSUES

o DYSBIOSIS: An imbalance of good and bad bacteria in the gut where the good bacteria decrease and bad bacteria increase. A gut test will reveal the level of Dysbiosis present in the gut. Dysbiosis symptoms can be diarrhoea, constipation, bloating, distension, abdominal pain/cramps, gas, losing the urge to poop, bad breath and an unpleasant odour from the colon when passing stool.

o SIBO (small intestinal bacterial overgrowth): this is a specific type of Dysbiosis diagnosed with a Hydrogen Breath Test costing £160 in 2020. The small intestine typically has a limited number of bacteria. SIBO occurs when excessive bacteria from other gut parts invade the small intestine. The symptoms of SIBO are like Dysbiosis and may include vomiting, diarrhoea, malnutrition, weight loss, and malabsorption.

o IBS: There is no specific test for IBS; however, a gut test will show what is wrong with your colon and may rule our other causes such as inflammatory bowel and coeliac disease.

TITBIT 15: WHAT IS POOP?

What is it made of?

Poop consists of 75 percent water and 25 percent solid matter. The solid matter consists of cellulose, dead bacteria, cholesterol, fats, calcium and iron phosphate, protein, cell debris shed from the mucous membrane of the intestinal tract, bile pigments (bilirubin), and dead leukocytes (white blood cells).

Why is it brown?

The brown colour is due to the action of bacteria on bilirubin which is the end product of the breakdown of haemoglobin (red blood cells).

Why does it smell?

The odour of poop comes from the chemicals produced by bacteria: indole, skatole, hydrogen sulphide, and mercaptans.

MY STORY: THE MICROBIOME AND GUT TESTS

I've mentioned my attempts to restore my gut health by eating soft, easily digestible food such as smoothies, soups, vegetables, and fruits. However, despite that, nothing had changed. I still didn't have an *urge to poop,* gas was still excessive, and the unpleasant odour when I pooped remained. Enemas were the only thing that helped me.

So, I had no other option but to order a gut test reluctantly (because of the cost). The test price varies, but mine cost £300 in 2020. Here's what the test included:

o My microbiome's health: stool consistency, pH levels, microbe diversity, enterotype, and Dysbiosis index.
o Bacteria, yeasts (including candida), moulds, parasites, and H. Pylori.
o Advanced gut health biomarkers: digestive function, immune system, and inflammation.

Other tests costing half this amount are available. Still, they only analyze the bacterial composition of the colon. They don't detect yeasts/candida, inflammation, moulds, parasites, and H. Pylori.

Getting a stool sample was challenging as you can't use an enema to poop because the water in the poop would affect the results. So, I took a hefty dose of an over-the-counter laxative for two days till I pooped. It was not a pleasant experience.

I posted the sample, and two weeks later, I received twelve pages of test results. Here's a summary of the Key Findings:

o A good stool PH.

o Good microbiome diversity.

o Moderate Dysbiosis. An imbalance of good and bad bacteria in the gut where the bad bacteria overpopulate the colon.

o Low levels of good bacteria: Bifidobacteria and Butyrate-producing bacteria.

o Elevated levels of potentially pathogenic (disease-causing) bacteria.

o Elevated levels of sulphate-reducing bacteria.

o A borderline positive result for the parasite Dientamoeba Fragilis.

o High secretory IgA (inflammation in the gut).

What I've written above is only a summary. The extensive report listed all the colon's microbes - bacteria, yeasts, moulds, and parasites. The report categorized the microbes into optimal (favourable) or out of range (unfavourable) and graded them as low, medium, or high. There were twenty-eight optimal microbes and twenty-four out of range. I intended to address the out-of-range microbes with probiotic supplements hoping this would restore the *urge to poop*.

I was grateful for the first two Key Findings, a good stool PH and a good microbiome diversity. These were probably due to eating fruits and vegetables all my life.

The thought of having a parasite shocked me, although I've since read that it's more common than people realize.

The last key finding, inflammation in the colon, can have many causes, such as an unhealthy diet, antibiotics, and Dysbiosis. It can also be hereditary or genetic, indicating that Inflammatory Bowel Disease (IBD) is developing. As my main focus is restoring the *urge to poop*, I'm hoping the level of inflammation will decrease when this happens. Interestingly an anti-inflammatory diet is similar to what I eat for constipation.

Here are the recommended supplements:
o Saccharomyces Boulardii, a probiotic (yeast) to support the gut-immune system.
o Clinical GI, a probiotic that features a bacteria strain and Bifidobacterium Lactis HNO19. Research has shown this improves 'whole gut transit,' meaning it may help alleviate constipation.
o Partially Hydrolysed Guar Gum (brand name Optifibre), a specific type of prebiotic fibre shown to support Butyrate-producing bacteria and may also help normalize bowel movements.
o Two anti-microbial oils, berberine and oregano, to help rebalance the microbiome.
o Cod liver oil – contains anti-inflammatory fats and Vitamin D and A. These are essential nutrients for a healthy microbiome, immune system, and gut lining.

I was to take the supplements for a minimum of eight weeks costing £380 in 2020. In the next My Story, you'll read my experience of taking the recommended products.

TITBIT 16: HOW TO POOP WITH MOO TO POO
There's a method for pooping called the Brace and Bulge, commonly known as Moo to Poo. It involves deep breathing while sitting on the toilet to relax your abdomen; then, with hands on your side, you say "M" and move your abdomen forward by adding "OO." This process opens the anal sphincter and helps relax the pelvic floor muscles, which enable the stool to pass. Search for this YouTube video with one and a half million views, "Natural Constipation Relief in 3 Easy Steps" (MOO to POO).

NOTE: the anal sphincter comprises two muscles at the end of the rectum. The muscles work together to keep stool in the rectum or eliminate stool from the body via a bowel movement.

9 Prebiotics and Probiotics

FACT FILE: PREBIOTICS AND PROBIOTICS

The global market for marketing probiotics is around fifty billion dollars a year and still growing. However, there's little marketing for prebiotics, because you can ingest them in cheap fibre supplements and food containing soluble fibre.

PREBIOTICS

o Prebiotics are compounds in food that feed probiotics, the good bacteria in the gut and help them flourish and multiply. They also prevent harmful bacteria from settling, which is vital for a healthy gut.

o You can ingest them in plant food with soluble fibre, such as apples, under-ripe bananas, onions, garlic, leek, asparagus, chicory, legumes, spinach, Jerusalem artichoke, carrots, flaxseeds/linseeds, and chia seeds. Resistant starch is also a prebiotic found in oats, lentils, rice, and potatoes. The resistant starch increases if the food is left to cool and reheated.

o Prebiotics can be taken in supplement form, although they may cause excess gas and bloating.

o Search on Amazon for prebiotic supplements and read the reviews. For example, inulin, made from chicory root, is widespread and inexpensive.

PROBIOTICS

- Probiotics are the good or friendly bacteria that live in our gut and benefit our gut health. We can ingest them in fermented food or as a supplement.
- Studies have shown they have several different functions: they help ensure the digestive system works correctly and that your body absorbs all the nutrients from your food; they help produce specific vitamins; break down fibre; expel bad bacteria and speed up stool transit time which is essential to prevent constipation.

WHAT YOU NEED TO KNOW ABOUT PROBIOTIC SUPPLEMENTS

- Manufacturers make probiotic supplements from freeze-dried bacteria, which thaw when absorbed by the body. However, studies have shown stomach acid kills sixty percent of most probiotic strains before reaching the colon. It's thought that probiotics need to have an enteric coating to be protected from stomach acid. Still, manufacturers of probiotics dispute this, saying stomach acid doesn't kill their probiotics so they don't need an enteric coating.
- Established bacteria (probiotics) living in the gut's mucous membrane resist new bacteria and prevent them from colonizing.
- When you stop taking probiotic supplements, the body loses the benefits within a few days. For this reason, you must take them daily to benefit the gut.
- Taking too many probiotics can cause nausea, bloating, and gas. People with weakened immune systems or severe illnesses should check with their doctor before taking them.

o It's uncertain if probiotics help SIBO sufferers (small intestinal bacterial overgrowth). However, studies have shown that Metronidazole/Fraygl, an antibiotic taken with Saccharomyces Boulardii, has a high success rate for treating SIBO.

WHAT SUPPLEMENTS TO BUY?

o Probiotics are measured in Colony Forming Units (CFUs). A high CFU count is needed to make an impact because of the sixty percent killed by stomach acid. The most effective probiotic supplements contain fifty billion CFUs.

o The best researched and commonly used strains of probiotics are Bifidobacterium, Lactobacillus, and Saccharomyces Boulardii, a yeast. The first two are more resistant to stomach acid than other probiotics, and the latter is resistant to antibiotics.

o The best probiotics contain between four to twelve strains of bacteria which can be beneficial in addressing certain physical conditions.

o The most effective strains for constipation are:
Bifidobacterium Lactis BB-12.
Bifidobacterium Lactis HN019.
Bifidobacterium Lactis DN-173 010
Lactobacillus Rhamnosus GG.

PROBIOTICS IN FERMENTED FOOD

o One of the richest sources of probiotics is cultured/fermented *homemade* food and drinks such as Yogurt, Sauerkraut, Kefir, Kimchi, and Kombucha.

o Manufacturing processes can kill the bacteria in food sold in supermarkets. As a result, the European Food

82

Safety Authority has banned the manufacturers of Yakult and Actimel from advertising that their food promotes health as no research supports these claims.

SOIL-BASED ORGANISMS (SBO FOR SHORT)

- Soil-Based Organisms are known as Spore Forming Probiotics.
- They are bacteria naturally found in soil that manufacturers use in probiotic supplements, health food, and health drinks.
- There are several reasons manufacturers like them: they form spores that can resist stomach acid and antibiotics; they survive the extreme heat used in food processing; they have a long shelf life, so they don't need refrigerated.
- They argue that our fruits and vegetables are squeaky clean compared to the past because of our modern farming methods. As a result, it's thought that our microbiome and immune system have lost the benefits they once had from ingesting SBOs in our food. They put forward the worldwide increase in allergies to support this argument.
- The argument against them is that they're soil bacteria not naturally found in our microbiome, so the body sees them as intruders in the gut. Spore-forming bacteria multiply rapidly: the concern is that they may take over the good bacteria in the gut and prove challenging to remove.

SYMPROVE

At present (2022) Symprove is only available in the UK. However, VSL#3 is a probiotic that, in some ways, is similar and available in the US. Symprove is a water-based food supplement with four strains of live, active bacteria. They recommend that 70 ml of Symprove is drunk every morning for twelve weeks to establish and colonize the bacteria in the gut. In 2015 University college London tested Symprove and confirmed that the bacteria in Symprove can *arrive, survive, and thrive in the gut* (quote from Symprove website). Check out their website for more information and reviews of people who've used it.

MUTAFLOR PROBIOTIC

In recent years scientists have studied Mutaflor more than any other probiotic worldwide. Research has shown it to be effective in treating Ulcerative Colitis, Chronic Constipation, and other gut issues. Professor Alfred Nissle of Germany discovered Mutaflor in 1917 during World War One. He was searching for bacteria that would inhibit the growth of intestinal pathogens and came across a soldier who, unlike other soldiers, hadn't contracted dysentery, typhoid fever, bacterial infections, or inflammation of the gut. So, professor Nissle isolated a unique E. coli strain from the stool of the soldier and developed Mutaflor.

The Mutaflor factory is in Germany, so their website is in German. The best place to get information is on their Australian website:
www.mutaflor.com.au.

In the UK, you can buy it from an online pharmacy:
www.breakspearmedical.com.

It's not available in the US but can be purchased from an online health store in Canada and shipped to the US: www.feelgoodnatural.com.

Mutaflor recommends you take their tablets for eight weeks, but they are expensive to buy. However, a YouTube video titled "How to Make Mutaflor Yogurt" by Josh Brown shows how to make three hundred Mutaflor capsules for £5, a fraction of the cost of the manufacturer's tablets.

There's also a doctor's website with instructions on making Mutaflor at home:
www.drmyhill.co.uk/wiki/Growing_Mutaflor

TITBIT 17: FECAL MICROBIAL TRANSPLANT (FMT)
An FMT is when a doctor transplants the faeces from a healthy donor into the bowel of a patient suffering from bowel disorders or diseases such as Clostridium Difficile (C. diff), Irritable Bowel Syndrome (IBS), Crohn's Disease, Ulcerative Colitis, Chronic Diarrhoea, and Constipation. A tube is inserted through the anus into the colon during the transplant, and the donor stool is released. The transplant aims to replace the good bacteria that antibiotics or other bad bacteria in the colon may have suppressed or killed. Search the Web to learn more about FMT, its high success rate, and how some people do their own FMT at home.

I left out the berberine and oregano oil to reduce the cost of the supplements recommended in my gut test results. I had great hope that what I was taking would be effective, but I was deeply disappointed when there was no change in bowel habits after two months. I'd heard a gastroenterologist say that if a supplement didn't work within two months, it would probably not work.

Then I read an article on the Web that recommended taking probiotic enemas, as one hundred percent rather than sixty percent of the probiotic will go into the colon. This was good news! Here's a link to an online article you may like to read about probiotic enemas: https://www.healthline.com/health/probiotic-enema#how-it's-done or search the Web for *probiotic enemas*.

Before taking the probiotic enema, you must clear the bowel first. I made the enema by emptying one capsule of Clinical GI probiotic into one cup of warm water, and I retained the enema for fifteen minutes. I took the enema in the morning and felt good after it; this could have been psychological or the effects of the probiotics. Either way, it didn't do me any harm. I took them weekly and then twice weekly as I'd read the body loses the benefits of probiotics in a few days and I thought this would be more effective. (I'm not recommending this, just sharing my experience.)

However, after two months of probiotic enemas and no change as far as I could tell, I stopped taking them. Once again, I was disappointed that the results I'd hoped for didn't happen. So, I switched focus to eating high-fibre food and consuming Kefir and Sauerkraut. I only eat homemade fermented food as manufacturing processes kill the bacteria in the food sold in supermarkets.

I read an article online about Soil Based Organisms. I ordered a two-month supply hoping again that this may be my cure, but sadly, nothing had changed at the end of the two months. Since then, I've read online articles against taking SBOs. Unfortunately, there are so many contradictions around supplements it's challenging to know what to take.

I wouldn't say I liked the thought of parasites in my body, and I'd read that if you restore your gut health, parasites will leave. That may be true, but I wanted to eliminate them if they exacerbated my constipation. So, I joined a few Facebook Parasite groups and discovered antibiotics, and herbal remedies may eliminate parasites depending on their type. However, I didn't go that route because antibiotics can kill good bacteria. Also, according to Facebook posts, herbal remedies could be expensive, time-consuming, and sometimes unsuccessful.

Then I heard about an American doctor, Jennifer Daniels, who recommends a parasite cure of turpentine (food grade pure pine spirit) and sugar cubes. You eat two sugar cubes saturated with turpentine in the morning for three days. I'm not recommending this; just sharing my experience. You'll need to conduct research on the Web for more information. After three mornings, the turpentine taste was repulsive, so I haven't tried it again. The parasite I tested positive for was

Dientamoeba Fragilis. Still, I have no idea if the cure worked as it's invisible to the human eye. Only another gut test will reveal if it worked, and I may repeat the treatment before I have another test. If you join a Parasite Facebook group, be careful, as some folks are obsessed with parasites, and it would be easy to get caught up with others in this obsession. Also, watch out for horrific photos!

I read about Symprove, a water-based food supplement containing four strains of bacteria that studies had shown had a positive effect on the gut. The reviews on their online community were positive, with many saying it had helped with constipation and IBS. So, I decided to take it for the recommended twelve weeks. I bought one month's supply and was delighted when they emailed me an offer to buy one month and get one month free near the end of my first month. Sadly, there was no change in constipation or change in the bad bacteria levels in my gut after twelve weeks.

I watched a YouTube video by Tony Grandov (the admin on the Facebook group Reversing Chronic Constipation Naturally) titled *The Miracle Probiotic that Cured my Constipation*. The miracle probiotic he was referring to was Mutaflor. So, I decided to try it, and there was a difference after two days. The poops were softer and better formed, more sausage-like than round balls; sorry if this is TMI (too much information). However, there was still no *urge to poop*, and I was still using enemas. So, I continued taking Mutaflor for the recommended eight weeks but no further changes. Once I stopped taking it, the softer, better-formed poops stopped.

Mutaflor is expensive, so I suggest taking one course for five days to see if it changes anything. Tony Grandov says Mutaflor cured his constipation in a few days, although he continued to take the entire course.

NOTE: I've just read on Tony Grandov's YouTube channel that, sadly some of his gut issues have slowly crept back since coming off Mutaflor.

TITBIT 18: THE GUT MICROBIOME
In the past ten years, there has been an explosion of scientific research on the gut microbiome. The research shows that the state of our gut can affect our risk of chronic disease: autoimmune reactions, allergies, food intolerance, mental health, obesity, and immune function (seventy percent of our immune system is in the gut). Eating fermented food is one of the best ways to help the gut. An American physician in alternative medicine, Dr. Joseph Mercola, sent his homemade Sauerkraut to a lab. He said, "We had it analyzed. We found ten trillion bacteria in a *4 to 6 ounce serving of the fermented vegetables." This far surpasses the probiotics you would get in the most expensive probiotic capsules (*114g to 170g).

10 Epilogue

It had been three years since I lost the *urge to poop,* and I had no idea what to try next. I was extremely disappointed that nothing I'd tried enabled me to poop without an enema.

However, I have a faith and have always prayed for help with constipation and, at times, received answers.

I have many examples of answered prayer; this is just one. In Chapter 3, My Story: Water, I write that several years ago, I had *bricklike* stools even though I was eating high-fibre food and drinking lots of water. So, I prayed about this, and it came to me that I drink copious cups of tea. I then googled, "Is tea constipating?" and discovered that caffeine in tea could be constipating. So, I switched to decaf tea, and within a few days, the *bricklike* stools softened.

So, I doubled my prayers on what to try next. Later that day, I remembered an online article I'd read by a gastroenterologist who said it might be challenging to eradicate bad bacteria when it invades the colon. I had a lightbulb moment and began to think *outside the box.* Then, I realized everything I'd read by gut experts said to feed the colon with good bacteria in food and supplements. They said this would colonize the colon with good bacteria and expel the bad bacteria, but this wasn't happening. So, it occurred to me that I needed something that would kill the bad bacteria rather than feed the good bacteria.

One of the results from my gut test showed that I had elevated levels of sulphate-reducing bacteria. So, I researched on the Web and discovered that sulphate-reducing bacteria can cause elevated levels of gas; the bacteria also help produce hydrogen sulphide, which participates in gut inflammation and has an unpleasant odour. This information convinced me that sulphate-reducing bacteria was the main problem in my colon. I had all the symptoms - excess gas, inflammation in the colon, and an unpleasant odour when I pooped.

So, I searched the Web for a remedy to kill sulphate-reducing bacteria. Then I found an article on how Lemongrass oil in enemas can kill these bacteria and how Epsom Salts baths put sulphate back in the body. Next, I read how to make the enema, ten drops of Lemongrass oil to one litre of water. Repeat this for seven days, and after the enema, soak in a hot water bath with one cup of Epsom Salts for thirty minutes. I was glad I noted the remedy as I could not find that article again.

So, in the morning, I took water enemas to clear my bowel, then I took the Lemongrass oil enema and retained it for twenty minutes. I followed this with an Epsom Salts bath. On the third day, I was so constipated that it took four water enemas back-to-back to clear my bowel. But on the fourth day, there was a massive improvement. The unpleasant odour was completely gone. My lower bowel emptied with only one water enema, and the excessive gas reduced significantly. The Lemongrass oil had killed the sulphate-reducing bacteria, which was an incredible breakthrough, although I still had no *urge to poop.*

However, over the next few months, the symptoms of bad bacteria returned twice – the unpleasant odour, a worsening of constipation, and excess gas, so I repeated the remedy. Both times, the Dysbiosis cleared, and six months later hasn't returned. Unfortunately, when I first took the remedy, I was a bit lazy and did it for four days and not the recommended seven, which could be why the bad bacteria grew again.

Then one morning, something incredible happened! I felt an *urge to poop*, and I pooped without an enema! However, it didn't happen every day, and there was some straining involved which I knew would lead to hemorrhoids. So, I decided to continue with water enemas on alternate days if I hadn't pooped naturally and focus on speeding up the transit time. But I was delighted to poop without an enema, even if only occasionally. At least I knew there was nothing physically wrong with my colon.

So, I prayed again and what came to me was to take three fibre supplements a day. I usually took two, one in the morning and one in the evening. However, instead of adding another fibre supplement drink I divided the three into two drinks. Since doing this, the *urge to poop* is getting stronger. It doesn't always lead to pooping naturally, but sometimes it does.

I've read many books on constipation and gut health. They tend to finish on a positive note, saying, "follow my seven-step plan, and you will poop regularly," or even worse, "follow my seven-step plan, and you will cure your constipation." However, I followed their plan, and nothing happened!

The positive note to end my book is to outline seven things that have helped me with constipation.

Help One: I discovered caffeine in tea and casein in cow's milk constipated me.

Help Two: Homemade soups and smoothies were an easy way to get enough fibre to help me poop.

Help Three: I learned that fermented homemade food such as Kefir and Sauerkraut feed the good bacteria in my colon more effectively than taking probiotic supplements.

Help Four: Through the finger-prick nutrition test, I discovered I was deficient in Vitamin D and borderline on Vitamin B12, which can exacerbate constipation.

Help Five: I discovered that coffee enemas clean my colon, detox my liver and give me a feeling of well-being. Also, a colonic can clear my colon of impactions or hard waste that could lead to an obstruction.

Help Six: The gut test, showed me exactly what was going on in my colon and what I needed to address. I had an imbalance of good and bad gut bacteria, with the bad bacteria overpopulating the colon (known as Dysbiosis). Low Levels of good bacteria and elevated levels of potentially pathogenic (disease-causing) bacteria. I also had a parasite and inflammation of the gut.

Help Seven: I discovered Lemongrass oil taken in an enema would kill the bad bacteria and that a remedy of food-grade turpentine and sugar cubes would kill parasites.

Interestingly what didn't help was the approximately £850 I spent on probiotics. I'm not saying probiotics wouldn't help others; I'm just saying they didn't help me. It could be that the sulphate-reducing bacteria had invaded my colon so much that probiotics had a negligible effect.

However, if I don't eat a diet high in fibre and drink lots of water daily, it's back to *bricklike* stools. So, all I'm doing is managing my constipation. The above *Helps* aren't a cure. I also find constipation frustrating because I think it's improving then for no reason that I can see its worsening! I know the root of my constipation is slow peristalsis, but I haven't found a remedy to quicken it. However, as I wrote earlier, I have a faith and will continue to pray and try any natural remedies I hear about that promise to quicken peristalsis or relieve constipation.

Thank you for buying my book and taking the time to read it. I hope you've learned something that will help you poop more regularly.

Blessings
Helen

An Amalgamation of My Story

1 My Story: Constipation

As a child, I grew up in a house in Scotland with eleven people: my mum, dad, five brothers, and three sisters. I didn't have a problem living with ten people. Still, I had a problem with only one bathroom in the house, as whenever I had *the urge to poop,* someone else in the family was using it. In addition, I was an introverted child in an extroverted family and didn't fight for my place in the queue.

From four years of age, I had frequent upset tummies. Finally, at seven years of age, I was rushed to the hospital for an operation to remove a suspected burst appendix. However, after the procedure, the surgeon said the cause of the stomach pain was constipation and not an infected appendix. So, every Sunday after church, my mum gave me a large tablespoon of a stimulant laxative, which meant I had a clear-out on Monday. She also fed me lots of fruit, and homemade soups full of vegetables and legumes, establishing a lifelong healthy eating habit for which I'm grateful. The laxatives and the fruits and vegetables helped me poop two or sometimes three times a week, but it was always with straining.

I have no recollection of pooping regularly in childhood. Then at school and later in the workplace, I was so embarrassed at how long I spent in the bathroom that I would *hold it in* and wait till I was home. I had no idea this was creating a problem in my intestines and would worsen my constipation in the long term.

In my mid-twenties, I had two children and, during the pregnancies, suffered severe constipation. I was prescribed laxatives which gave temporary relief, but I knew it wasn't a long-term solution. In my thirties, I read many books on constipation, looking for the root cause and what I could do about it. I learned about *withholding* or *resisting the urge to poop,* which can begin early in life when a child is embarrassed to use public bathrooms or doesn't like the *smelly* school bathrooms. I had a lightbulb moment as I read this and realized that when I was a child and had the *urge to poop,* but someone was using the family bathroom, I would *withhold.* Then at school, because I took so long in the bathroom, I withheld again till I was home to avoid embarrassment.

With more reading, I learned that when we eat, the muscles in the walls of our gut contract and relax. As a result, the food is moved forward in a wavelength motion known as peristalsis, which gives us the *urge to poop.* I resisted this urge by *withholding,* and through time those muscles weakened, resulting in slow transit constipation. Fast forward to March 2019, when I lost the *urge to poop.* I'm certain it was caused by eating a low-carb diet for a year which you'll read about in Chapter 7, My Story. The scary thing about it was that nothing I'd done in the past to manage my constipation helped me with this new difficulty of having no *urge to poop.*

I was four years old when constipation started, and at the time of writing this (2022), I'm now sixty-nine. That's sixty-five years! It's incredible that the world can send a man to the moon but can't come up with a cure for constipation.

2 My Story: Dietary Fibre

Constipation was a significant problem by the time I was thirty; I pooped once or twice a week and strained to pass incredibly hard stool. That was when I took laxatives which worked erratically. I was concerned about their long-term use and if they would harm my body. However, if I didn't take them, I worried about all the stool stuck in my colon and the painful hemorrhoids caused by straining. Eventually, I stopped taking laxatives and have recently read many posts on Facebook groups where members write that, in time, laxatives became ineffective in helping them poop. In addition, they caused irreversible damage to the colon in some people.

I noticed that I pooped more frequently if I ate high-fibre food. So, the bulk of my diet became vegetables, fruit, legumes (beans, peas, lentils, chickpeas), wholegrains such as oats, barley, wholemeal bread and wholewheat pasta. It was challenging to follow a vegetarian diet because I cooked for my family, so I settled on less meat with more vegetables for my evening meal.

However, I needed discipline to eat high-fibre food and resist processed food. When I was sick, emotionally upset, on holiday, or celebrating, I lost that discipline and went days without pooping – I'm only human!

At this point, I resorted to a water enema rather than a laxative to clear my colon and returned to eating lots of high-fibre food. During this time, I began tracking my food to ensure I was eating enough fibre and drinking adequate water to manage constipation. Until I was sixty-five, this regime worked for me, and I could poop two or sometimes three times a week, depending on how much water and fibre I consumed.

Fast forward to March 2018, when I ate a low-carb diet for health reasons. Eating adequate fibre on a low-carb diet isn't easy, so I began taking two fibre supplements each day. I had one after breakfast and one after dinner, which was 7g daily. So along with the 23g of fibre I ate in my food, I ate 30g daily. However, low-carb vegetables have very little soluble fibre, so stool was often hard and difficult to pass. By March 2019, I was chronically constipated, and lost the *urge to poop*. I resorted to water enemas to have a bowel movement but was concerned that the enemas were ineffective some days. In the end, I decided to come off the low-carb diet and return to a diet high in soluble fibre. However, *gas* became so bad that I was nervous about leaving the house, and I still couldn't poop without a water enema. The only benefit was that the water enemas worked well when I ate high-fibre food.

I used a notebook to track my food to determine which food was causing the gas. The worst culprits were legumes: beans, peas, and lentils, which I ate in my homemade soups, and oats which I had most mornings for breakfast. However, I was concerned it would be challenging to eat enough fibre if I cut out the food causing gas. For example, a bowl of porridge was 6g of fibre, and a bowl of my homemade soup was between 6g-10g of fibre. All I could do was avoid eating legumes and oats before being in the company of other people. I also discovered smoothies at this time, and if I couldn't have homemade soup or oats because I would be with other people, I had smoothies that are easy to digest, high in fibre, and cause much less gas.

I read many articles on the Web about gut health and learned about the gut microbiome and the importance of increasing the good bacteria in my gut. I experimented with fermented food, which has zero or little fibre but is full of good bacteria. I make Kefir all year and Sauerkraut only in the summer as I find it cold and unappealing in the winter. Water and coffee enemas became a big part of my regime, which I write about in Chapter 6.

There was one improvement. Homemade soups and smoothies gave less *bricklike* stool with water enemas. However, there was still no *urge to poop*, and I depended on enemas to clear my colon. Despite my efforts, I decided that there wasn't much improvement, and I needed something more. The something more was a Gut Test by Stool Analysis which you'll read about in Chapter 8.

3 My Story: Water

I've always been a Tea Jenny. I drank copious cups of tea every day, unconcerned about it as I'd read that tea could be included in my water intake. Then a few years ago, I read research on the Web that said tea, coffee, and cola are diuretics (because of the caffeine) and flush fluids out of the body, resulting in constipation.

Learning this was a eureka moment for me as I'd been drinking lots of caffeinated green tea for its health benefits throughout the day. However, an online article referred to it as *green tea constipation,* so I switched to decaffeinated green tea, and my stools became less *bricklike.* Another tea I like is Redbush tea or Rooibos, made from a South African herb, which I think is the only herbal tea that comes close to the taste of *real* tea. If you're concerned about tannins in tea, then Rooibos tea is an excellent choice as it's low in tannins. However, I like the buzz I get from a cup of caffeinated tea, so I allow myself one weak tea in the morning and one when I eat out.

HERE'S HOW I DRINK WATER
o I tracked my daily water intake and discovered the quantity that worked for me was a minimum of one and a half litres a day. If I had less than this, it was back to *bricklike* stools. I aim for two litres a day, but I don't consistently achieve this.

- I start drinking water as soon as I'm awake and aim for one litre in the morning. If I don't do this, it's challenging to reach my daily quota. Also, I don't drink in the evening to avoid trips to the bathroom during the night.
- I drink room temperature or hot water as it feels gentler on my insides than chilled water.
- Many health experts say not to drink liquid with a meal as it's not good for digestion. However, I ignore this and have a glass of squash/cordial with each meal. It's an effortless way to ensure I'm drinking enough water.
- I've always consumed hot water with lemon juice in the mornings, and I added Apple Cider Vinegar for a time. My recipe was ½ tablespoon lemon juice and ½ tablespoon ACV in 250ml water. However, after a while, I realized I wasn't drinking as much because I wasn't fond of the taste of ACV in the water, so I reverted to hot water and lemon juice.
- Most days, I drink one litre of plain water, and the rest is in decaf tea, soups, and diluting drinks such as squash or cordial.

4 My Story: Nutritional Supplements

After I stopped taking laxatives, I tried many vitamins, minerals, herbs, and enzymes. I spent considerable money on them, hoping to find a cure for my constipation. However, after several years without any change in constipation, I stopped everything except Vitamin C and Magnesium.

Over the years, I'd used a Vitamin C flush to cleanse the bowel by taking a 1000 mg tablet every hour for six hours till I pooped. Based on this experience, I decided to take two 1000 mg tablets daily, one in the morning and one in the evening, the recommended dose to help with constipation.

At the beginning of my year of eating low-carb, I experienced painful muscle cramps in my legs during the night. I posted on a Facebook group asking for advice, and a member replied to supplement with Magnesium. I was taking a low dose of Magnesium, but once I increased it, the cramps stopped. I was then confident that supplementing with Magnesium was effective. Muscle cramps are common on low-carb diets, as they exclude many high-carb foods containing Magnesium. It's said that most of the population in the Western world is deficient in Magnesium which is possibly why the recommended daily dosage of 400 mg for men and 320 mg for women seems high.

I read on the Web that deficiencies in Vitamin B12 and Vitamin D can cause constipation. I then discovered that a simple finger-prick blood test could reveal whether the body was deficient in these vitamins. So, I purchased a Nutrition Test Kit online, which would test for Magnesium, Vitamin B12, Vitamin D, inflammation, cholesterol, and triglyceride levels. It cost £80 in 2022, and I also paid £30 to have blood taken for the test at a clinic as I can never get enough blood with a finger-prick.

My results came in a few days later. They revealed that Magnesium levels were normal, probably because I take a Magnesium supplement. However, I was deficient in Vitamin D and borderline low in Vitamin B12. So, I started taking a daily Vitamin D supplement of 4000 IU (International Units). After that, I considered having a Vitamin B12 injection costing £30 and lasting six months (excess B12 is stored in the liver). However, I decided instead to eat liver once a fortnight, giving me a regular intake of B12.

I may retake the Nutrition Test in the future to check if things have changed for the better. The test also showed my HDL cholesterol was normal, but LDL cholesterol was too high, so I'm addressing this with my diet. I'd say the blood test was worthwhile, and I'm hopeful that, taking Vitamin D supplements along with eating liver for B12 will help with constipation in the long-term.

Regarding enzymes, I drink goat's milk all year and eat Sauerkraut in the summer. Both are high in enzymes.

5 My Story: Exercise

In my twenties and thirties, exercise was part of my life. I did a bit of jogging and worked out at the gym, but it did not affect my constipation. I exercise now by doing half an hour of walking outdoors and fifteen minutes of gentle resistance exercise several times a week. However, my reasons for doing this are more for general health than to help with constipation.

I had read the information on the Web about vibration. So, as I thought it might help, I bought a hand-held, battery-operated massage gun. I used it to massage the area over my colon, thinking it might speed up peristalsis. Unfortunately, I have wear and tear on my hands, and I found it difficult to hold and move the gun over my abdomen for more than 5 minutes. So, after several weeks, I stopped using it; however, I think it might work for some people if they could sustain its use for 15 minutes.

When I was reading about the Mowoot and vibration machines, I was interested but at the same time cynical about them working. Years of trying things that did not affect my constipation have made me like this! I don't want to spend a lot of money on something that may not be effective. It's good that the manufacturer gives a guarantee of a refund if it doesn't work but as it's delivered from Spain it could be complicated to return. I may look for a gym with a vibration machine and try that instead.

Another option is a vibration belt such as Slendertone, used to tone the abdominal muscles. I might consider asking for a vibration belt for Christmas or my birthday, and if it doesn't work for constipation, it may give me abs!

No doubt, like yourself, I get weary of everything I have to do for constipation, such as eating high-fibre food, drinking water, and taking enemas. However, I think a vibrating belt or machine promoting pooping could be the answer, although it would depend on the cost. I'm hopeful of the vibrating pill that may be for sale soon, and I will be trying that.

6 My Story: Enemas

I began taking water enemas over thirty-five years ago when I stopped taking laxatives. I read a book on constipation by a doctor who wrote that taking water enemas was preferable to taking laxatives or straining to poop as both may harm the body. So, if I hadn't pooped for a few days because I'd been eating processed food and not drinking enough water, I took a water enema to clear my bowel instead of a laxative. It was like starting again, and I immediately got back on track with high-fibre food and water.

If I left it longer than a few days, the stool became *bricklike,* and the water enema was ineffective. When this happened, I took a soap-suds enema and did two or three enemas back-to-back till my bowel was clear. In the years before my colon shut down, the frequency of pooping would be anything from thirty-six to seventy-two hours. I want to stress that I did not take regular daily enemas; I only took an enema if I'd gone more than sixty hours without pooping which could be once every few weeks. When I lost the *urge to poop* after following a low-carb diet, I took water and coffee enemas daily for four months, then switched to alternate days because of the time involved.

It was awkward and uncomfortable lying on the bathroom floor when I began to take frequent enemas. Then, I read a

Facebook post that suggested using pillows inside plastic bin liners, making it a much more comfortable experience.

Although I've read on the Web that you can retain a water enema for thirty minutes, I only retain them for fifteen minutes. My experience is that if they're not effective in the first fifteen minutes, they won't be effective after that. So, if the enema doesn't work, I use a fresh warm enema solution with liquid soap.

I had a friend of eighty-four who fell and broke her hip and was admitted to the hospital for a hip replacement. She also suffered from chronic constipation and was unable to poop after her operation. The hospital gave her large doses of laxatives over two days till her bowels moved. Unfortunately, she didn't make it from the bed to the bathroom. She said the mess on the floor and the foul odour was horrendous, and she was so humiliated by the experience that she couldn't stop crying. I would hate to experience that, and I'm grateful I discovered enemas.

For over thirty-five years, enemas have helped me avoid straining to pass *bricklike* stool, which can lead to hemorrhoids and anal fissures. I suffered from painful hemorrhoids before taking enemas but not since then.

I watched a YouTube video, and someone mentioned that coffee enemas could restore good bowel tone and improve peristalsis. However, I didn't find any research that confirmed this, but it got my attention. So, after conducting a Web search, I began taking daily coffee enemas in July 2019. They're for detoxing the liver (the largest organ in the body), improving health, stimulating the intestines, promoting bowel movements, and cleansing the colon. Initially, I didn't want to do coffee enemas as I was a bit nervous about putting *coffee up my butt*; it seemed a bit mad. However, the Facebook group *Coffee Enema Support* gave me the support and information I needed to get started.

So, what was my experience with coffee enemas? Once I saw the benefits of cleansing my colon and the feeling of well-being after the coffee enema (the effects of the caffeine), I decided to continue with them long-term. However, as the enema is retained for fifteen minutes to cleanse the liver of toxins, you must empty the bowel first. So, I had to take one or two water enemas before the coffee enema, which meant setting aside an hour in the morning to do this.

Around this time, I made three purchases. The first was a red rubber/latex catheter to replace the plastic nozzle on the enema tubing, a game-changer for comfort. The second was an electric water distiller to give me peace of mind that I wasn't filling my colon with contaminants from the water. Before this, I used boiled tap water. My third purchase was a Squatty Potty which I found effective.

The main benefit of taking coffee enemas was that the unpleasant odour from my colon decreased in the first week. Over the months, some odd stuff appeared in the stool, dislodged from the colon wall. So, the cleansing side worked, although I didn't notice any difference in transit time or frequency of pooping. I recently read that coffee enemas can improve peristalsis if taken for two years;

however, the article didn't quote any research to support this. After four months of daily coffee enemas, I switched to alternate days because of the time involved.

ENEMA BAG OR BUCKET?

For decades when I took an occasional enema, I used a plastic enema bag, easily purchased from pharmacies or on the Web and simple to use. You can hang them on the bathroom door handle or the toilet paper holder. They're easy to pack in a suitcase for holidays. Then, when I took coffee enemas, I switched to a metal bucket. I'd read that coffee can form mould in an enema bag's seams if not cleaned thoroughly.

However, one drawback with the metal bucket is that you can't see the liquid reducing (you can see it in a plastic bag or transparent plastic bucket). Another drawback in using the bucket for coffee enemas is that it's difficult for the last bit of liquid to flow out because of the tubing position. The problem with this is that the phytonutrients in the coffee can settle at the bottom of the bucket. However, if you can reach the bucket, it can be tipped slightly, so the liquid enters the tube, although my attempts at this have sometimes resulted in tipping the coffee over myself.

COLONIC IRRIGATION

After taking coffee enemas daily for four months, I visited a Colon Therapist for colonic irrigation, which involves flushing waste material out of the colon using a large amount of water. I'd read that coffee enemas can dislodge old waste material on the colon walls, and colonics can remove this. Then, after the colonic, the therapist told me that a hard piece of waste had come out, which she said may have caused a blockage in the future.

The colonic released a vast amount of waste, and for the first time in my life, I experienced an empty colon, and I felt ten-pound lighter! The only discomfort was slight stomach cramps just before my body expelled the waste. Also, I felt physically tired and drained after it, but this passed after a good night's sleep.

From my experience and the experiences of others on Facebook groups, I'd say that a colonic clears the bowel and may remove blockages but doesn't do anything for constipation in the long term. I would have a colonic in the future if I thought I had a bowel blockage or a bowel impaction. Overall, I'd say the colonic was a good experience, and I recommend them for having a clear-out.

7 My Story: Low-Carb Constipation

Many people eating low-carb have successfully lost excess weight and improved their health worldwide. I'm all for low-carb eating and in no way want to condemn it. What I've written here is simply my story of the effect low-carb eating had on my constipation.

From March 2018, for one year, I followed a low-carb Ketogenic Diet, Keto for short, with carbs limited to 20g a day. I have an autoimmune disease that causes swollen, painful joints. In only six weeks, the inflammation and the soreness lessened quite a bit. As well as this, I experienced a massive boost in energy, increased mental clarity, decreased cravings for sweet food, and a great night's sleep. A bonus was a seven-pound weight loss, so naturally, I was delighted!

When I began eating Keto, I was amazed to have regular soft poops; this was the only time I can remember this happening in my life. Sadly, after several weeks they stopped. There are two reasons why this may have occurred, but they are merely speculation.

First, the high fat in my diet, which was seventy percent of my total calories, may have caused the soft poops. Then my body may have adapted to the high fat and reverted to its constipated state. Second, the regular pooping may have stopped because I switched from what's known as *Strictly*

Keto to *Easy Keto*. I started having artificial sweeteners and low-carb food with additives such as colours, flavour enhancers, emulsifiers, stabilizers, and preservatives. As I explained in the Fact File, a *well-formulated keto diet* (WFKD) keeps the body in a constant state of ketosis. The liver then produces beta-hydroxybutyrate, which replaces some dietary fibre functions. So, introducing artificial sweeteners and additives may have lowered my body's ketosis. Then the liver stopped making beta-hydroxybutyrate, and regular pooping ceased.

So, with a return of constipation, I had to rise to the challenge of eating 30g of fibre a day while eating only 20g of carbs. I used a food tracker and included as many low-carb/high-fibre foods as possible to keep my fibre intake high. After breakfast and dinner, I took a fibre supplement, giving an additional 7g of fibre. This strategy worked for ten months apart from my usual bouts of constipation because I hadn't eaten enough fibre or drunk enough water. However, severe constipation kicked in towards the end of my year of eating Keto.

Pooping became less frequent; an unpleasant odour appeared on my breath and a more pungent odour from my colon when I pooped. Then, suddenly my bowels stopped working, and I lost the *urge to poop*. Finally, I resorted to daily water enemas to clear me out, but I had to have multiple enemas some days, which concerned me. I loved eating low carb because of the energy and health improvements. Still, I decided my colon health was more important, and reluctantly one year after I started, I gave up low-carb eating. I returned to how I previously ate, all fruits and vegetables, legumes, wholemeal bread, and wholewheat pasta, so there was an immediate increase in fibre, especially soluble fibre. The enemas were then effective, which relieved me, but I still had no *urge to poop.*

From reading on the Web, I discovered that low-carb eating could cause the good bacteria in the colon to die off, and the bad bacteria then multiply and overpopulate the bowel. I also read another online article about the role of the appendix in the body; remember, I had mine removed at age seven. I'd always read the appendix was a useless organ, but research now shows its role is to store good bacteria. If the colon becomes overpopulated with bad bacteria, the appendix releases its good bacteria to rebalance the colon. Discovering this information was another light bulb moment. I realized that my body couldn't address the imbalance in good and bad bacteria without an appendix, which was probably the cause of losing the *urge to poop.*

So, having learned this, my focus became repopulating the good bacteria in my colon through probiotics in food and supplements, which you'll read about in the following chapters.

8 My Story: The Microbiome and Gut Tests

I've mentioned my attempts to restore my gut health by eating soft, easily digestible food such as smoothies, soups, vegetables, and fruits. However, despite that, nothing had changed. I still didn't have an *urge to poop,* gas was still excessive, and the unpleasant odour when I pooped remained. Enemas were the only thing that helped me.

So, I had no other option but to order a gut test reluctantly (because of the cost). The test price varies, but mine cost £300 in 2020. Here's what the test included:

o   My microbiome's health: stool consistency, pH levels, microbe diversity, enterotype, and Dysbiosis index.

o   Bacteria, yeasts (including candida), moulds, parasites, and H. Pylori.

o   Advanced gut health biomarkers – digestive function, immune system, and inflammation.

Other tests costing half this amount are available. Still, they only analyze the bacterial composition of the colon. They don't detect yeasts/candida, inflammation, molds, parasites, and H. Pylori.

Getting a stool sample was challenging as you can't use an enema to poop because the water in the poop would affect the results. So, I took a hefty dose of an over-the-counter laxative for two days till I pooped. It was not a pleasant experience.

I posted the sample, and two weeks later, I received twelve pages of test results. Here's a summary of the Key Findings:

o   A good stool PH.
o   Good microbiome diversity.
o   Moderate Dysbiosis. An imbalance of good and bad bacteria in the gut where the bad bacteria overpopulate the colon.
o   Low levels of good bacteria: Bifidobacteria and Butyrate-producing bacteria.
o   Elevated levels of potentially pathogenic (disease-causing) bacteria.
o   Elevated levels of sulphate-reducing bacteria.
o   A borderline positive result for the parasite Dientamoeba Fragilis.
o   High secretory IgA (inflammation in the gut).

What I've written above is only a summary. The extensive report listed all the colon's microbes - bacteria, yeasts, moulds, and parasites. The report categorized the microbes into optimal (favourable) or out of range (unfavourable) and graded them as low, medium, or high. There were twenty-eight optimal microbes and twenty-four out of range. I intended to address the out-of-range microbes with probiotic supplements hoping this would restore the *urge to poop.*

I was grateful for the first two Key Findings, a good stool PH and a good microbiome diversity. These were probably due to eating fruits and vegetables all my life.

The thought of having a parasite shocked me, although I've since read that it's more common than people realize.

The last key finding, inflammation in the colon, can have many causes such as an unhealthy diet, antibiotics, and Dysbiosis. It can also be hereditary or genetic, indicating that Inflammatory Bowel Disease (IBD) is developing. As my main focus is restoring the *urge to poop*, I'm hoping the level of inflammation will decrease when this happens. Interestingly an anti-inflammatory diet is similar to what I eat for constipation.

Here are the recommended supplements:
o Saccharomyces Boulardii, a probiotic (yeast) to support the gut-immune system.
o Clinical GI, a probiotic that features a bacteria strain and Bifidobacterium Lactis HNO19. Research has shown this improves 'whole gut transit,' meaning it may help alleviate constipation.
o Partially Hydrolysed Guar Gum (brand name Optifibre), a specific type of prebiotic fibre shown to support Butyrate-producing bacteria and may also help normalize bowel movements.
o Two anti-microbial oils, berberine and oregano, to help rebalance the microbiome.
o Cod liver oil – contains anti-inflammatory fats and Vitamin D and A. These are essential nutrients for a healthy microbiome, immune system, and gut lining. I was to take the supplements for a minimum of eight weeks costing £380 in 2020. In the next My Story, you'll read my experience of taking the recommended products.

9 My Story: Probiotics and Prebiotics

I left out the berberine and oregano oil to reduce the cost of the supplements recommended in my gut test results. I had great hope that what I was taking would be effective, but I was deeply disappointed when there was no change in bowel habits after two months. I'd heard a gastroenterologist say that if a supplement didn't work within two months, it would probably not work.

Then I read an article on the Web that recommended taking probiotic enemas, as one hundred percent rather than sixty percent of the probiotic will go into the colon. This was good news! Here's a link to an online article you may like to read about probiotic enemas: https://www.healthline.com/health/probiotic-enema#how-it's-done or search the Web for *probiotic enemas.*

Before taking the probiotic enema, the bowel must be cleared first. I made the enema by emptying one capsule of Clinical GI probiotic into one cup of warm water, and I retained the enema for fifteen minutes. I took the enema in the morning and felt good after it; this could have been psychological or the effects of the probiotics. Either way, it didn't do me any harm. I took them weekly and then twice weekly as I'd read the body loses the benefits of probiotics in a few days and thought this would be more effective. (I'm not recommending this, just sharing my experience.)

However, after two months of probiotic enemas and no change as far as I could tell, I stopped taking them. Once again, I was disappointed that the results I'd hoped for didn't happen. So, I switched focus to eating high-fibre food and consuming Kefir and Sauerkraut. I only eat homemade fermented food as manufacturing processes kill the bacteria in the food sold in supermarkets.

I read an article online about Soil Based Organisms. I ordered a two-month supply hoping again that this may be my cure, but sadly, nothing had changed at the end of the two months. Since then, I've read online articles against taking SBOs. Unfortunately, there are so many contradictions around supplements it's challenging to know what to take.

I wouldn't say I liked the thought of parasites in my body, and I'd read that if you restore your gut health, parasites will leave. That may be true, but I wanted to eliminate them if they exacerbated my constipation. So, I joined a few Facebook Parasite groups and discovered antibiotics, and herbal remedies may eliminate parasites depending on their type. However, I didn't go that route because antibiotics can kill good bacteria. Also, according to Facebook posts, herbal remedies could be expensive, time-consuming, and sometimes unsuccessful.

Then I heard about an American doctor, Jennifer Daniels, who recommends a parasite cure of turpentine (food grade pure pine spirit) and sugar cubes. You eat two sugar cubes saturated with turpentine in the morning for three days. I'm not recommending this; just sharing my experience. You'll need to conduct research on the Web for more information. After three mornings, the turpentine taste was repulsive, so I haven't tried it again. The parasite I tested positive for was Dientamoeba Fragilis. Still, I have no idea if the cure worked as it's invisible to the human eye. Only another gut test will reveal if it worked, and I may repeat the treatment before I have another test. If you join a Parasite Facebook group, be careful, as some folks are obsessed with parasites, and it would be easy to get caught up in this obsession. Also, watch out for horrific photos!

I read about Symprove, a water-based food supplement containing four strains of bacteria that studies had shown had a positive effect on the gut. The reviews on their online community were positive, with many saying it had helped with constipation and IBS. So, I decided to take it for the recommended twelve weeks. I bought one month's supply and was delighted when they emailed me an offer to buy one month and get one month free near the end of my first month. Sadly, there was no change in constipation or change in the bad bacteria levels in my gut after twelve weeks.

I watched a YouTube video by Tony Grandov (the admin on the Facebook group Reversing Chronic Constipation Naturally) titled *The Miracle Probiotic that Cured my Constipation*. The miracle probiotic he was referring to was Mutaflor. So, I decided to try it, and there was a difference after two days. The poops were softer and better formed, more sausage-like than round balls; sorry if this is TMI (too much information). However, there was still no *urge to poop, and I was still using enemas.* So, I continued taking

121

Mutaflor for the recommended eight weeks but no further changes. Once I stopped taking it, the softer, better-formed poops stopped.

Mutaflor is expensive, so I suggest taking one course for five days to see if it changes anything. Tony Grandov says Mutaflor cured his constipation in a few days, although he continued to take the entire course.

NOTE: I've just read on Tony Grandov's YouTube channel that, sadly some of his gut issues have slowly crept back since coming off Mutaflor.

10 Epilogue

It had been three years since I lost the *urge to poop,* and I had no idea what to try next. I was extremely disappointed that nothing I'd tried enabled me to poop without an enema. However, I have a faith and have always prayed for help with constipation and, at times, received answers.

I have many examples of answered prayer; this is just one. I write in Chapter 3, My Story: Water, that several years ago, I had *bricklike* stools even though I was eating high-fibre food and drinking lots of water. So, I prayed about this, and it came to me that I drink copious cups of tea. I then googled, "Is tea constipating?" and discovered that caffeine in tea could be constipating. So, I switched to decaf tea, and within a few days, the *bricklike* stools softened.

So, I doubled my prayers on what to try next. Later that day, I remembered an online article I'd read by a gastroenterologist who said it might be challenging to eradicate bad bacteria when it invades the colon. I had a lightbulb moment and began to think *outside the box.* Then, I realized everything I'd read by gut experts said to feed the colon with good bacteria in food and supplements. They said this would colonize the colon with good bacteria and expel the bad bacteria, but this wasn't happening. So, it occurred to me that I needed something that would kill the bad bacteria rather than feed the good bacteria.

One of the results from my gut test showed that I had elevated levels of sulphate-reducing bacteria. So, I researched on the Web and discovered that sulphate-reducing bacteria could cause elevated levels of gas; the bacteria also help produce hydrogen sulphide, which is involved in gut inflammation and has an unpleasant odour. This information convinced me that sulphate-reducing bacteria was the main problem in my colon. I had all the symptoms - excess gas, inflammation in the colon, and an unpleasant odour when I pooped.

So, I searched the Web for a remedy to kill sulphate-reducing bacteria. Then I found an article on how Lemongrass oil in enemas can kill these bacteria and how Epsom Salts baths put sulphate back in the body. Next, I read how to make the enema, ten drops of Lemongrass oil to one litre of water. Repeat this for seven days, and after the enema, soak in a hot water bath with one cup of Epsom Salts for thirty minutes. I was glad I noted the remedy as I could not find that article again.

So, in the morning, I took water enemas to clear my bowel, then I took the Lemongrass oil enema and retained it for twenty minutes. I followed this with an Epsom Salts bath. On the third day, I was so constipated that it took four water enemas back-to-back to clear my bowel. But on the fourth day, there was a massive improvement. The unpleasant odour was completely gone. My lower bowel emptied with only one water enema, and the excessive gas reduced significantly. The Lemongrass oil had killed the sulphate-reducing bacteria, which was an incredible breakthrough, although I still had no *urge to poop.*

However, over the next few months, the symptoms of bad bacteria returned twice – the unpleasant odour, a worsening of constipation, and excess gas, so I repeated the remedy. Both times, the Dysbiosis cleared, and six months later hasn't returned. Unfortunately, when I first took the remedy, I was a bit lazy and only did it for four days and not the recommended seven, which could be why the bad bacteria grew again.

Then one morning, something incredible happened! I felt an *urge to poop*, and I pooped without an enema! However, it didn't happen every day, and there was some straining involved which I knew would lead to hemorrhoids. So, I decided to continue with water enemas on alternate days if I hadn't pooped naturally and focus on speeding up the transit time. But I was delighted to poop without an enema, even if only occasionally. At least I knew there was nothing physically wrong with my colon.

So, I prayed again and what came to me was to take three fibre supplements a day. I usually took two, one in the morning and one in the evening. However, I divided the three into two drinks instead of adding another fibre supplement drink. Since doing this, the *urge to poop* is getting stronger. It doesn't always lead to pooping naturally, but sometimes it does.

I've read many books on constipation and gut health. They tend to finish on a positive note, saying, "follow my seven-step plan, and you will poop regularly," or even worse, "follow my seven-step plan, and you will cure your constipation." However, I followed their plan, and nothing happened!

The positive note to end my book is to outline seven things that have helped me with constipation.

Help One: I discovered caffeine in tea and casein in cow's milk constipated me.

Help Two: Homemade soups and smoothies were an easy way to get enough fibre to help me poop.

Help Three: I learned that fermented homemade food such as Kefir and Sauerkraut feed the good bacteria in my colon more effectively than taking probiotic supplements.

Help Four: Through the finger-prick nutritional test, I discovered I was deficient in Vitamin D and borderline on Vitamin B12, which can exacerbate constipation.

Help Five: I discovered that coffee enemas clean my colon, detox my liver, and give me a feeling of well-being. Also, a colonic can clear my colon of impactions or hard waste that could lead to an obstruction.

Help Six: The gut test, showed me exactly what was going on in my colon and what I needed to address. I had an imbalance of good and bad gut bacteria, with the bad bacteria overpopulating the colon (known as Dysbiosis). Low Levels of good bacteria and elevated levels of potentially pathogenic (disease-causing) bacteria. I also had a parasite and inflammation of the gut.

Help Seven: I discovered Lemongrass oil taken in an enema would kill the bad bacteria and that a remedy of food-grade turpentine and sugar cubes would kill parasites.

Interestingly what didn't help was the approximately £850 I spent on probiotics. I'm not saying probiotics wouldn't help others; I'm just saying they didn't help me. It could be that the sulphate-reducing bacteria had invaded my colon so much that probiotics had a negligible effect.

However, if I don't eat a diet high in fibre and drink lots of water daily, it's back to *bricklike* stools. So, all I'm doing is managing my constipation. The above *Helps* aren't a cure. I also find constipation frustrating because I think it's improving then for no reason that I can see its worsening!

I know the root of my constipation is slow peristalsis, but I haven't found a remedy to quicken it. However, as I wrote earlier, I have a faith and will continue to pray and try any natural remedies I hear about that promise to quicken peristalsis or relieve constipation.

Thank you for buying my book and taking the time to read it. I hope you've learned something that will help you poop more regularly.

Blessings
Helen

Book 2 – It's All About The Food

This short book is my follow-up to Help! I
Can't Poop! and in it, I share everything
I've learned about which foods to
eat and avoid to help you poop!

I'ts All About The Food

Copyright and Disclaimer

Table of Contents

Notes For The Reader

MEASUREMENTS
The measurements used in the recipes and the listings for fruits and vegetables are European Metric and US Imperial.

WORD CHOICE AND SPELLING
o   The word *gas* rather than *wind* is used for flatulence.
o   The UK and US differ in the spelling of certain words. The UK spelling *fibre* is used rather than the US spelling *fiber*.

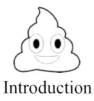

Introduction

You may have read my first book, *Help! I Can't Poop,* where I write about everything that has helped me in my journey with constipation for over sixty years. A significant step in my journey has been learning which foods helped me poop or worsened my constipation. So, the focus of this book is food.

It has information that will help you choose the food to eat and avoid to help you poop. For example, it has the fibre content for popular fruits and vegetables, lists food and drinks to help you poop, gives examples of how to calculate the fibre in your food, and lists the food that may be exacerbating your constipation or causing digestive distress.

My favourite part of the book is Chapter 4, *How to Use a Food Tracker.* Using a Tracker is the key to discovering which foods help you with constipation and which foods exacerbate it. It's a simple tool that can affect how often you poop.

Enjoy a Coffee, and a Fruit Muffin for your mid-morning snack, or if you're eating low-carb, have a Flaxseed Biscuit. Recipes are in Chapter Seven.

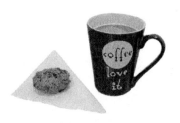

Bon Appetite!
Helen

1 Foods That May Constipate You

Many people find they have a sensitivity or intolerance to a particular food, which can exacerbate constipation, so they eliminate that food from their diet. Here's a list of the most common ones.

○ Milk and dairy products contain lactose, a type of sugar found in milk. Suppose your body isn't producing enough of the enzyme lactase to digest lactose. Then, the lactose will cause gas, bloating, constipation, and diarrhea, known as lactose intolerance.

○ Milk contains the protein casein, which some people find binding and constipating. Any dairy food made with milk from animals would have the same effect.

○ Wheat, barley, and rye products contain the protein gluten. The most common symptom of gluten intolerance or sensitivity to gluten is bloating.

○ Legumes (beans, peas, lentils, chickpeas) have a carbohydrate known as raffinose which the body cannot digest and
  may cause gas and bloating.

NOTE: on Facebook groups, some members post that when they eliminated either dairy, gluten, or legumes from their diet, their constipation lessened and, in some cases eradicated.

The first time I drank my homemade Kefir I pooped the next day; sadly, this never happened again. The following day I was terribly constipated. I posted on a Facebook group, and a member responded that it would be the casein in cow's milk and switch to goat's milk. Goat's milk contains casein, but it's less dense than cow's milk and many people tolerate it better than cow's milk. It also has less lactose than cow's milk, so people who are intolerant or sensitive to casein and lactose do better on goat's milk. A way to check if cow's milk is constipating you is to drink at least one cup a day for a few days and see if it affects your bowel movements. If it does, do the same thing with goat's milk to see if there's any difference.

LOW FODMAP DIET

FODMAP stands for fermentable oligosaccharides, disaccharides, monosaccharides, and polyols. These are short-chain carbohydrates (sugars) that the small intestine absorbs poorly. As a result, some people experience digestive distress after eating them.

o Monash University in Australia developed the diet to help sufferers of IBS. It's an elimination diet where you cut out all high FODMAP food, food high in certain sugars that cause digestive distress. You can then gradually reintroduce them to discover which food triggers symptoms.

o The diet addresses symptoms such as gas and bloating but doesn't address the underlying cause of the digestive distress. In addition, it's not meant to be followed long-term as much of the eliminated food contains soluble fibre, and the lack of this may worsen the underlying cause.

o High FODMAP food includes wheat products, dairy, legumes, artificial sweeteners, vegetables such as onions, asparagus, artichokes, garlic, and fruit such as pears, apples, peaches, and cherries. You can find more information at the Monash University website: www.monashfodmap.com and you can also download the FODMAP App.

TIPS ON REDUCING GAS CAUSED BY LEGUMES

An indigestible carbohydrate called raffinose causes the gas in beans. The body doesn't digest raffinose, and bacteria in the bowel break it down, producing gas. Raffinose is also in cruciferous vegetables, but other compounds in these vegetables can cause gas. Lentils are a high-fibre and high FODMAP food, so they can be a trigger food for gas in many people. Here are some tips to reduce gas from legumes.

- o First, soak in cold water for at least 24 hours and rinse well before cooking.
- o Add one teaspoon of bicarbonate of soda to the soaking water.
- o Add one teaspoon of the Mexican herb Epazote to the legumes while cooking.
- o Beano is a food supplement that comes in tablet form. The marketing says, "containing a natural food enzyme that breaks down the complex sugars found in many foods, making them easier to digest so they don't cause gas." You take it just before you eat.

FOOD LACKING IN FIBRE AND NUTRITION

Food made by manufacturers is known as processed food, such as plain yogurt or wholemeal bread. However, food manufactured with sugar, unhealthy fats, and additives such as sweeteners, colouring, stabilizers, and preservatives become ultra-processed food.

o Ultra-processed food lacks fibre and nutritional value, yet now makes up over 50% of the UK and US diet.

o Unfortunately, these foods can also taste delicious, such as cakes, biscuits, sweets, chocolate, breakfast cereals, and take-away food. As a result, you may need a transition from eating ultra-processed food to eating whole fresh food rich in fibre to help you poop.

THE SHOCKING TRUTH ABOUT VEGETABLE OILS

Vegetable oils such as rapeseed, sunflower, safflower, corn, canola, and sesame are loaded with polyunsaturated fats. These fats are unstable and can cause intestinal problems such as leaky gut syndrome and immune system disorders. In addition, they're linked to cancer, heart disease, arthritis, obesity, and type 2 diabetes. A better name would be Industrial Seed Oil, as they're not made from vegetables but extracted from seeds.

They've only existed since the early 1900s, when new industrial processes could extract high volumes of oil from the seeds. The oil produced is a disgusting dark, sticky, smelly substance that's then processed to produce oils and spreads (margarine) that look and taste edible. The process involves the use of chemicals and bleaching and deodorizing. After this process, the oils are devoid of nutrients or antioxidants but leave pesticides untouched. It's then advertised as a healthy product! Replace vegetable oils and spreads with butter, olive oil, avocado oil, and beef tallow/dripping.

2 Food and Drink to Help You Poop

Here's a list of food other than popular fruits and vegetables to help increase your fibre intake. The list isn't exhaustive as there are other high-fibre foods. Also, the food marked with an asterisk are suitable for low-carb eaters.

*AVOCADO: 100g has 6.7g of fibre, 4oz has 7.7g of fibre. It's packed with fibre and is excellent in salads or smoothies.

BAKED BEANS: 100g has 3.7g of fibre, 4oz has 4.2g of fibre. Beans are an easy and tasty way to increase fibre intake. You can eat them on wholemeal toast, baked potato, or as a side vegetable.

BAKED POTATO: 100g has 2.5g of fibre, 4oz of raw potato with the skin before baking has 2.8g of fibre. It can be eaten for lunch or dinner and topped with baked beans or chili to increase the fibre.

*CHIA SEEDS: one tablespoon or 13g has 4g of fibre. It takes on the flavour of the food it's added to, such as soup, cereal, smoothies, or yogurt. Chia seeds are best pre-soaked for 30 minutes before eating.

Chia seeds and flaxseeds/linseeds contain a helpful fibre known as mucilaginous fibre. This type of fibre forms a gel during the digestive process when it mixes with water, soothing inflamed tissue in the gut lining.

*FLAXSEEDS/LINSEEDS: 8g or one tablespoon has 2g of fibre. You can add the seeds to porridge, homemade muesli, or soup. Eat ground flaxseeds, as whole flaxseeds pass through the body undigested and don't have any health benefits. Ensure you drink lots of water when eating flaxseed.

LEGUMES: beans, peas, lentils, and chickpeas are all legumes. When cooked, 100g has 5g of fibre, 4oz has 6g of fibre, but check the manufacturers packaging for the exact amount of fibre. As well as being high in fibre legumes are high in protein and carbohydrates but low in fat.

*NUTS: they're high in fibre and calories, so you may only want to eat a small amount. Here's the fibre in 30g/1oz of popular nuts: almonds 2.2g; brazil 2.2g; cashew 2g; coconut 3.4g; hazelnut 2.9g; macadamia 2.5g; peanuts 2.5g; pecan 2.9g; pine 1g; pistachio 1g; walnut 2g.

PASTA AND RICE: wholewheat pasta has 4.5g of fibre per 100g, 5.5g of fibre per 4oz. Brown rice has 2g of fibre per 100g, 2.4g of fibre per 4oz. Please refer to the manufacturer's nutrition label on the packaging for the exact fibre content. The wholewheat or brown versions of these foods are high in fibre. So, try including them in your evening meals with bolognaise or curries.

Sir William Arbuthnot Lane was a surgeon in the early 1900s who specialized in colorectal surgery. In his retirement, he toured Europe and gave lectures about the benefits of fruits, vegetables, sunshine, and exercise on our health. He believed disease could be prevented by developing certain habits and said, "The whiter your bread, the sooner you're dead."

PEAS: 100g has 5g of fibre, 4oz has 5.8g of fibre. Eat them as a side vegetable or on their own with salt and pepper.

PORRIDGE: a serving of 30g/1oz or has 2.7g of fibre. Add bran, flaxseeds, or chia seeds to increase the fibre content.

PRUNES (dried plums): a serving of 50g has 3.5g of fibre, 2oz has 4g of fibre. As well as being high in fibre, prunes contain the natural laxative sorbitol. It acts as a mild colonic stimulant that reduces stool transit time.

*SEEDS (other than flaxseeds and chia seeds): seeds like nuts can be high in fibre and calories. Here's the approximate fibre in 30g/1oz of some popular seeds: hemp 2g; pumpkin 2g; sesame 3.5g; sunflower 1.8g.

WHEAT BRAN: a serving of two-level tablespoons or 7g has 3g of fibre. When wheat is processed, the outer layer becomes a by-product called bran. Add to porridge for breakfast.

WHOLEMEAL BREAD: an average serving of one slice has 2.9g of fibre (this differs depending on the brand and size of the slice). Bread can be toasted and topped with beans for a high-fibre lunch.

DRINKS TO HELP YOU POOP

Drink these remedies on an empty stomach first thing in the morning.

PRUNE JUICE

Drink one-half to one cup of prune juice. Warm juice is more effective on the colon.

WATER AND LEMON JUICE WITH APPLE CIDER VINEGAR

Sip one litre of hot water with two tablespoons of lemon juice and two tablespoons of apple cider vinegar (ACV is optional). For a smaller early morning drink, use 250ml/8oz water with half a tablespoon of lemon juice and half a tablespoon of apple cider vinegar.

WATER AND LEMON JUICE FOLLOWED BY PRUNE JUICE

Sip one litre of hot water with two tablespoons of lemon juice and follow it with one cup of prune juice.

CHIA SEED TEA

Make one cup of tea with 250ml/8oz water and your favorite tea: green, black, herb, or flavoured. Let the tea cool slightly before adding the seeds to avoid clumping together. Next, add one level tablespoon of chia seeds and stir well. The tea can be drunk hot or chilled. An option is to add ½ tablespoon of lemon juice. Also, to get the full benefits of the chia seeds, leave the tea for 20 minutes and then reheat if desired.

CELERY JUICE

You will need an electric juicer to make this. A juicer separates juice and fibre in food, leaving all the nutrients in the liquid. Then, within minutes of drinking, the nutrients are in our bloodstream.

Although there is no fibre in celery juice, it is high in mannitol, a type of sugar alcohol. It acts as an osmotic, pulls water into your colon, and loosens stool.

One large batch of celery will make approximately sixteen fluid ounces or ½ litre of juice.

3 Does the Time we Eat Matter?

Does it matter when we eat if we can't poop? According to science, the answer is yes.

Your body has a mechanism known as the Migrating Motor Complex (MMC), which, if working well, can help you poop more regularly.

MMC stimulates peristalsis, the wave-like muscle contraction in the walls of the colon, which moves food along and eventually eliminates it from the body.

An impaired MMC will cause slow peristalsis leading to constipation. However, MMC switches off while you're eating or digesting food and only works between meals, during fasting, and when you are asleep.

It can take several hours for the body to work through the MMC cycle; therefore, space your meals a minimum of four hours apart and, if possible, practice overnight fasting for a minimum of twelve hours. This limited eating time would mean no all-day snacking or midnight feasts!

Many people practice Intermittent Fasting (IF), which is simply having a period of eating food, followed by a period of abstaining from food. IF is described by two numbers, such as 16/8, the popular protocol, 16 hours fasting with an 8-hour eating window. For example, the fast might begin at

6 pm, and you break it at 10 am the following morning. Although you may prefer 12/12, 12 hours fasting, and 12 hours eating, which would still benefit the MMC and stimulate peristalsis and hopefully more regular pooping.

Conduct a Web search to discover the many health benefits of practicing Intermittent Fasting.

If you decide to practice either spaced-out meals or fasting, ensure you have plenty of water and fibre when you eat and drink.

4 How to Use a Food Tracker

A *Food Tracker* is a paper tool to help you on your journey with constipation. Each day you track what you're consuming: the food you eat, the amount of fibre, water intake, nutritional supplements, and whether you've pooped. Then, from day two, you can make adjustments according to what has worked or not worked for you, and you can repeat this as often as you like.

You may like to try a One-Day Tracker (ODT), where you record in a notebook everything you eat in a day with a note of the fibre. The tracker is simply a tool to give you an idea of how much fibre you're eating, whether 15g or 25g, and how your body reacts to it.

After a while, tracking becomes easier as we mostly eat the same foods, and you'll get to know the fibre content. Also, if you buy a bag of oranges approximately the same size, work out the fibre for one orange and use that amount for all the oranges in the bag. You can do this with any multiple foods you buy. Here are three examples of Food Trackers. The fibre amount has been rounded up or down to '0.5' or '0' to make it easy to calculate.

One Day Tracker - Thursday 5th March

Breakfast	
½ cup of Kefir	0
Recipe 3 Porridge	7g
Lunch	
Recipe 6. Thai Sweet Potato Soup	8.5g
Wholemeal Bread & Butter	2.5g
Dinner	
Chicken Breast	0
Potatoes 120g/4oz	2.5g
Broccoli 120g/4oz	3g
Snacks	
Chopped apple 150g/5oz	3.5g
Recipe 18 Flaxseed Biscuit / Butter	3.5g
Total Fibre	30.5g
Total water	2L
Vitamin C and D; Magnesium.	√√√
Pooped	10 am

Notes
A lot of gas from the soup.

One Day Tracker – Friday 6th March

Breakfast	
½ cup of Kefir	0
Recipe 14 Raspberry Smoothie	10g
Lunch	
Sandwich with meat and salad	2.5g
Dinner	
*Recipe 5. Easy-Peasy Soup	10.5g
MacDonalds Burger & Fries	3.5g
Snacks	
Large Orange	4g
Total Fibre	30.5g
Total water	2 L
Vitamin C and D; Magnesium	√√√
Pooped	None
Notes	
Soup before MacDonalds works!	

One Day Tracker–Saturday 7thMarch

Breakfast	
½ cup of Kefir	0
Wholemeal Toast, Butter	2.5g
1½ Fibre Supplements	5.5g
Lunch	
Scrambled egg	
Wholemeal toast, butter	2.5g
Dinner	
Sausages	
Mash Potato 150g/5oz	3.5g
Baked Beans 100g/3.5oz	3.5g
1½ Fibre Supplements	5.5g
Snacks	
Apple 5oz/150g	3.5g
Total Fibre	28.5g
Total water	1.5L
Vitamin C & D, Magnesium	√√√
Pooped	2 pm
Notes	
Grateful for fibre supplements.	

5 Calculating the Fibre in Food

To calculate the fibre content in fruits and vegetables, you can download a phone app from the Apple App Store or Google Play. Two popular Apps are My Fitness Pal and Carb Manager. These apps have a database of millions of foods with accurate nutrition facts. You input your food and its weight, and it will calculate the value of the fibre as well as fat, protein, carbs, and calories.

However, you can also work out the fibre using a calculator. Refer to the lists of fruits and vegetables in Chapter 6 for their fibre content. Here are some examples of metric and imperial weight.

METRIC
100g of apple has 2.4g of fibre (from the list in Chapter 6)
If you've eaten 145g of apple, your calculation would be like this:
145g ÷ 100g x 2.4g = 3.5g
So 145g apple has 3.5g of fibre

100g of broccoli has 2.6g of fibre (from the list Chapter 6).
If you've eaten 80g of broccoli, your calculation would be like this:
80g ÷ 100g x 2.6g = 2.08g
So 80g of broccoli has approximately 2g of fibre.

European packaged food manufacturers mainly calculate the nutritional information from 100g, but there are exceptions. So, for example, the nutritional information on packaged lentils may say 80g of lentils has 8.5g of fibre.

If you've eaten 60g of lentils, your calculation would be like this:

60g ÷ 80g x 8.5g = 6.37g

So 60g of lentils contain 6.3g of fibre

IMPERIAL

4oz of apple has 2.7g of fibre (from the list in Chapter 6).

If you've eaten 5oz of apple, your calculation would be like this:

5oz ÷ 4oz x 2.7g = 3.37g

So 5oz of apple has 3.3g of fibre

4oz of broccoli has 3g of fibre (from the list in Chapter 6). If you've eaten 3oz of broccoli, your calculation would be like this: 3 oz ÷ 4oz x 3g = 2.25g

So 3oz of broccoli has approximately 2.2g of fibre

If you're calculating the fibre in packaged food, do this:

For example, the nutrition label on packaged lentils may say 3oz of raw lentils has 9g of fibre. If you've cooked 2oz of raw lentils, your calculation would be like this:

2oz ÷ 3oz x 9g = 6g

So 2oz of raw lentils has 6g of fibre.

6 Fibre Content in Fruits and Vegetables

This chapter is simply a list of the fibre content in popular fruits and vegetables. Knowing how much fibre is in these foods will help you work out how much or how little fibre you're eating.

The first number following the fruit is fibre per 100g, and the second number is fibre per 4oz.

Apple 2.4g/2.7g
Apricot flesh 2g/2.3g
Avocado flesh 6.7g/7.6g
Banana flesh 2.6g/2.9g
Blackberry 5.3g/6.5g
Blueberry 2.4g/2.7g
Cherry plus stone 2.1g/2.4g
Clementine flesh 1.7g/1.9g
Coconut flesh 9g/10.2g
Date flesh 7.5g/8.5g
Elderberry 7g/7.9g
Fig 2.9g/3.3g
Gooseberry 4.3g/4.9g
Grapefruit 1.6g/1.8g
Grape 0.9g/1g
Guava 5.4g/6.1g
Kiwifruit 3g/3.4g
Kumquat 6.5g/7.3g
Lemon flesh 2.8g/3.2g

Lime flesh 2.8g/3.2g
Loganberry 5.3g/6g
Mango 1.6g/1.8g
Melon Cantaloupe flesh 0.9g/1g
Melon Honeydew flesh 0.8g/0.9g
Melon Watermelon 0.4g/0.5g
Mulberry 1.7g/1.9g
Nectarine with stone 1.7g/1.9g
Olives, pitted 3.3g/3.7g
Orange flesh 2.4g/2.7g
Papaya flesh (Paw Paw) 1.7g/1.9g
Passion Fruit flesh 10.4g/11.8g
Peach with stone 1.5/1.7g
Pear with core 3.1g/3.5g
Persimmon 3.6g/4.1g
Pineapple flesh 1.4g/1.6g
Plum with stone 1.4g/1.6g
Pomegranate flesh 4g/4.5g
Quince 1.9g/2.1g
Raspberry 6.5g/7.3g
Rhubarb 1.8g/2g
Satsuma flesh 1.3g/1.5g
Strawberry 2g/2.3g

Kiwi has an enzyme called actinidin. Studies have shown that eating two peeled kiwi fruit per day is an effective treatment option for constipation. Some people also eat the edible skin.

Pineapple has an enzyme called bromelain that helps bowel function and controls regularity.

Plums contain the natural laxative sorbitol, a mild colonic stimulant that reduces stool transit time.

Rhubarb is considered a natural laxative and has been used through the centuries to relieve constipation.

The first number following the vegetable is per 100g, and the second number is per 4oz.

Artichoke 5.4g/6.1g
Asparagus 2g/2.4g
Aubergine 3.0g/3.4g
Bean Sprouts 2g/2.3g
Beets 2.8g/3.2g
Beetroot 2.8g/3.2g
Broccoli 2.6g/2.9g
Brussel Sprouts 3.8/4.3g
Butternut Squash 2.0g/2.3g
Cabbage 2.5g/2.8g
Cauliflower 3.0g/3.6g
Carrots 2.8g/3.2g
Celeriac 1.8g/2g
Celery 1.6g/1.8g
Cucumber Unpeeled 0.5g/0.6g
Green Beans fine 2.7g/3.1g
Kale 3.6g/4.1g
Leek 1.8g/2g
Lettuce 1.3g/1.5g
Mushrooms 1g/1.1g
Mustard Greens 1.7g/1.9g
Onions 1.7g/1.9g
Okra 3.2g/3.6g

Parsley 3.3g/3.7g

Parsnip 4.9g/5.5g

Peas, garden 5.7g/6.4

Peas, sugar snap 2.6g/2.9g

Peppers, green 1.7g/1.9g

Peppers, red 2.1g/2.4g

Peppers, yellow 9g/1g

Potato 2.5g/2.8g

Pumpkin 0.5g/0.6g

Radish 1.6g/1.8g

Shallots 3.2g/3.6g

Spaghetti Squash 1.5g/1.7g

Spinach 2.2g/2.5g

Swede 2.3g/2.6g

Sweet Potato 3.0g/3.4g

Sweet Corn 2.0g/2.3g

Tomatoes 1.2g/1.4g

Turnip 1.8g/2g

Zucchini (Courgettes) 1g/1.1g

7 Recipes

I've read many recipes for constipation in books and on the Web. Still, I haven't tried many, mainly because the ingredients can cost a small fortune. Also, recipes for a healthy gut seem to be full of food I dislike, such as tofu and kale, and I find when I eat food I dislike, it can lead me to binge on chocolate. Then there's the food I've never seen in my local supermarket in Scotland, such as Napa cabbage or Shiitake mushrooms.

So, I developed recipes based on the food I enjoyed rather than what others recommended. I started by listing the food I liked and created meals, soups, smoothies, and snacks. I eat very simply and plainly, and don't use a lot of herbs and spices; however, I'm sure you could take my recipes and jazz them up a bit with seasonings.

NOTES ON RECIPES
Some of the recipes use coconut drink or coconut milk. Fresh coconut drink comes in cartons, and you can find it in the supermarket's refrigerated section, or if it's *long-life*, it's stored on the shelves. Coconut milk comes in cans and is thicker, creamier, and fattening!

Measurements are in metric and imperial, and where it's a cup or spoon, it's always a level measurement.

Cornflour is known as cornstarch in the US.

INDEX OF RECIPES

1) MUESLI FOR ONE
Total 7g of fibre per serving.

Ingredients
45g/1½oz porridge oats, fibre 4g
1 tbsp/8g ground flaxseed, fibre 2.2g
1 tbsp/7g flaked almonds, fibre 0.5g
1 tbsp/12g sultanas or raisins, fibre 0.4g

Put all the ingredients into a cereal bowl, stir and add milk
of your choice.
****

2) LOW-CARB MUESLI FOR ONE
Total 4g of fibre and 2.2g of carbs per serving.
If you're struggling to reach your fat macros, this recipe has
22g of healthy fats.

Ingredients
4 tsp/10g flaxseed, fibre 2.2g and carbs 0.2g
1½tbsp/10g flaked almonds, fibre 0.7g and carbs 0.7g
2 tbsp/10g flaked coconut, fibre 1.2g and carbs 0.6g
½ tsp sweetener
2 tbsp almond milk
2 tbsp single cream, carbs 0.7g

Put all the dry ingredients into a bowl and stir to combine.
Mix the milk and cream and pour over the muesli. Don't
leave the liquid in the muesli for more than a few minutes,
as it will thicken and won't have the consistency of milk.
****

3) PORRIDGE FOR ONE
Total 7g of fibre per serving.

Ingredients
45g/1½oz porridge oats, fibre 4g
250ml/8oz water
2 tbsp/7g wheat bran, fibre 3g
Put the porridge and the water into a small pot and cook till
simmering. Turn the heat down and continue cooking while

stirring for a few minutes. Add the two tablespoons of wheat bran and cook and stir for a few more minutes. Pour into a bowl and add milk and sugar/sweetener if desired. NOTE: you can replace wheat bran with one tablespoon of flaxseed, 2.2g of fibre.

****

HOMEMADE SOUPS
Here are five soup recipes, three with added beans that increase the fibre content. I use canned Navy/Haricot beans and drain the liquid before using, but you can use any canned beans or chickpeas. You can also strain and wash canned baked beans and add these to the soup. However, the beans are optional, and you can omit them from the recipes. To thicken the soup, use cornflour (cornstarch in the US) or use arrowroot, potato starch, or a small amount of guar gum.

4) LENTIL SOUP FOR FOUR
Total 40.3g of fibre without beans for the whole recipe. Add 11.2g of fibre if beans are included or 6.3g of fibre if potatoes are added.
The recipe makes approximately 1900 ml/2 quarts of soup.

Ingredients
240g/8oz red lentils, fibre 30.8g
180g/6oz carrots, fibre 5.2g
180g/6oz onions, fibre 4.3g
2 tbsp cornflour
400g/14oz can navy/haricot beans, fibre 11.2g
OR
540g/20oz can potatoes, fibre 6.3g

3 ham or vegetable stock cubes
1500ml/3 US pints (50oz) cold water

NOTE: weigh the onions and carrots after chopping and grating. The potatoes are an alternative to the beans. If the liquid in the soup reduces in cooking, add some stock at the end to replace it.

If using cans of beans or potatoes, drain the liquid and chop the potatoes. Set aside till later. Grate the carrots and finely chop the onions. Put the lentils, carrots, onions, and stock cubes into a large pot. Put the cornflour in a cup with a bit of cold water and stir to form a paste. Bring the soup to a boil, add the cornflour and the cooked beans or potatoes, then simmer for 35 minutes. Stir the soup frequently as lentils easily stick to the bottom of the pot.

You can also make this soup in a slow cooker/crockpot, and there's less danger of the lentils sticking to the pot. To reduce the time the soup takes to boil, use boiling water from a kettle rather than cold water. Set the slow cooker on high until it boils, turn to low, and simmer for an hour.
****

5) EASY-PEASY SOUP FOR ONE
Total 7g of fibre for the recipe without beans and 10.4g of fibre with beans.
You can make this soup with frozen mixed vegetables or fresh vegetables. For the beans, you can strain and wash canned baked beans.

Ingredients

180g/6oz mixed vegetables, fibre 7g
60g/2oz cooked beans, fibre 3.4g
½ stock cube
1½ cups cold water
1 tsp (optional) cornflour

Put the water into a pot. Crumble the stock into the water and add the vegetables and beans. Stir the cornflour into a little cold water to form a paste, add to the water, and stir. Bring to the boil and simmer for 5 minutes. The soup can be eaten with whole vegetables or blended to make a delicious smooth soup. Alternatively, blend the vegetables, then add the beans. Potatoes can be used instead of beans and you can increase the number of ingredients to make a larger volume of soup.
****

6) THAI SWEET POTATO SOUP

Total 33.6g of fibre for the whole recipe without beans and 43.7g with beans.
The recipe makes approximately 2.4 litres/2.5 quarts of soup. A blender is needed to make a smooth soup. Most ingredients are frozen or canned, but if using fresh vegetables, weigh after peeling. Once you cook the vegetables, put the mixture into the blender.

Ingredients
900g/21oz sweet potato, fibre 24.3g
180g/6oz chopped onion, fibre 3.1g
600ml/20oz coconut drink
¾ Tbsp Thai red curry paste
345g/20oz cooked potatoes, fibre 6.2g

240g/8oz cooked beans, fibre 13.4g
2 stock cubes
1000ml/2 US pints (34oz) of cold water

Put all the ingredients except the beans and the coconut drink into a large pot. Bring to boil and simmer for 30 minutes. Stir with a wooden spoon to prevent the mixture from sticking to the bottom of the pot. Pour the soup into a blender and blend till smooth. Drain the beans and add them with the coconut drink to the soup. Heat gently as heating rapidly, impairs the flavour of the coconut drink. You can also make the soup in a slow cooker/crockpot. Once the soup is boiling, lower the temperature and simmer until the vegetables are cooked. Transfer to a blender, then back to the pot, add the beans and coconut drink, and heat gently.
****

7) SCOTCH BROTH FOR FOUR
Total 34.5g of fibre.
The recipe makes approximately 1900 ml/2 quarts of soup.
Soak the broth mix overnight in a bowl of cold water. The next day, put the broth mix in a cauldron and rinse thoroughly under cold running water.

Ingredients
60g/2oz barley, fibre 10.4g
30g/1oz red lentils, fibre 3.3g
90g/3oz dried marrowfat peas, fibre 12g
120g/4oz chopped leeks, fibre 2.0g
150g/5oz/carrots, grated. fibre 4.3g
150g/5ozturnip, grated, fibre 2.5g
3 chicken/vegetable stock cubes

162

2 tbsp cornflour with a bit of water
1.5 litres/3.2 US pints (51oz) water

NOTE: instead of leeks, you can use onions, and instead of turnip, use parsnip. Weigh vegetables after peeling. You can use frozen or fresh leeks. If the liquid in the soup reduces in cooking, add stock at the end to replace it.

Put all the ingredients (except the cornflour) into the soup pot and bring to a boil. Next, simmer the soup for at least one hour, stirring occasionally. Then, mix the cornflour with a bit of cold water in a cup to form a paste. Add to the soup, stir well, and cook for 10 minutes. Alternatively, put all the ingredients into a slow cooker/crockpot and cook for around 6 hours. To cook quicker, use boiled water from a kettle. Cook on high till simmering, then continue to cook for one hour.

****

8) LOW-CARB BROCCOLI & CAULIFLOWER SOUP FOR ONE

Total 5.6g of fibre and 5g of carbs per serving.
The recipe will make a bowl of thick and rich-tasting soup.
Double or triple the ingredients to make more portions.

Ingredients
120g/4oz broccoli, fibre 2.9g and carbs 2.6g
120g/4oz/ cauliflower, fibre 3.6g and carbs 3g
1 tbsp double cream, carbs 0.2g
¾ cup/185ml stock or broth
Add seasoning.

Cook frozen or fresh veg in a pot till tender. Use an immersion hand blender to blend the vegetables. Add the cream, stock, and seasoning. Stir well and heat to serve. An option is to add 30g/1oz of grated cheese and simmer and stir till the cheese is melted. The grated cheese can also rest on top of the soup. Another option is to add chopped ham, chicken, or chopped/crumbled bacon.

****

9) LOW-CARB LUNCHTIME SALAD FOR ONE
Total 5.5g of fibre and 4g of carbs per serving.

Ingredients
1 serving of protein: chicken, cheese, egg, or meat.
45g/1½oz chopped tomatoes, fibre 0.54g. and carbs 0.8g
45g/1½oz chopped mushrooms, fibre 0.45g and carbs 0.9g
15g/½oz green pitted olives, fibre 0.5g and carbs 0.1g
60g/2oz avocado, fibre 4g and carbs 1.1g
2 tbsp/30g mayonnaise, carbs 1.1g

Chop all the ingredients, put them in a bowl, add mayonnaise, and mix well. Other low-carb salad vegetables are celery, cucumbers, lettuce, and peppers.

****

The following recipes are chickpea curry and sweet and sour vegetables using manufactured sauces. They're easy to make and tasty!

10) PLANT-BASED CHICKPEA CURRY FOR TWO
Total 11.9g fibre for one serving.

The vegetables can be stir-fried first in oil, but this is optional. Weigh vegetables after chopping.

Ingredients
240g/8oz can of chickpeas, fibre 9.8g
210g/7oz mushrooms, fibre 2.0g
210g/7oz onions, fibre 3.3g
210g/7oz cauliflower, fibre 6.3g
120g/4oz red pepper, fibre 2.4
1 Jar curry sauce, check manufacturer's label for fibre

Cut the stalks off the cauliflower and cut the flower part into small bite-sized chunks. Next, chop the mushrooms and onions and put all the vegetables into a wok or pot on the hob. Then, add the sauce and stir and simmer for 15 minutes. Serve with brown rice and wholewheat nan bread. These will increase the fibre content.
****

11) PLANT-BASED SWEET AND SOUR VEGETABLES FOR TWO
Total of 10.3g of fibre for one serving. The vegetables can be stir-fried first in oil, but this is optional. Weigh vegetables after chopping.

Ingredients
210g/7oz mushrooms, fibre 2g
210g/7oz onions, fibre 3.3g
120g/14oz red pepper, fibre 2.4g
225g/1 8oz can bamboo shoots, fibre 1.7g
225g/1 8oz can water chestnuts, fibre 1.8g

1 Jar sweet & sour sauce, check manufacturer's label for fibre

Chop the mushrooms, onions, and pepper and put them in a wok or pot on the hob. Next, add the drained bamboo shoots and water chestnuts. Then, stir the ingredients and add the sauce. Bring to a boil and simmer for 15 minutes. Serve with brown rice and prawn crackers. The rice will increase the fibre content.
****

12) PLANT-BASED CHILI FOR TWO
Total 14.2g of fibre per serving.
The vegetables can be stir-fried first in oil, but this is optional. Weigh vegetables after chopping.

Ingredients
400g/14oz can tomatoes, fibre 6g
400g/14oz can kidney beans, fibre 14.8g
210g/7oz mushrooms, fibre 2.0g
210g/7oz onions, fibre 3.3g
120g/4oz red pepper, fibre 2.4
2 tbsp tomato paste
1 vegetable stock cube
50ml/¼ cup boiled water
*1 teaspoon chili powder
1 tablespoon cornflour with a bit of cold water
*If you're not used to chili, start with ½ tsp

Chop the mushrooms, onions, and peppers, and put them in a deep frying pan or pot on the hob. Add the can of chopped tomatoes with the liquid, the drained beans, tomato paste, and chili powder. Dissolve the stock cube in the boiled water and stir into the vegetables. Put the cornflour in a cup, add a bit of cold water, and stir. Add to the vegetables and stir and simmer for 15 minutes. Serve with brown rice, wholewheat wraps, or baked potato, which will increase the fibre content.

****

13) STIR-FRIED CABBAGE FOR ONE
Total 9.5g of fibre per serving.

Ingredients
Use frozen or fresh cabbage.
210g/7oz cabbage, fibre 4.9g
120g/4oz onions, fibre 1.9g
1 large apple, fibre 2.7g
1 or 2 tbsp olive oil
Seasoning: salt, white pepper, cumin
Note: an option is to add some chopped fried bacon.
Chop the cabbage if it's fresh and not frozen. Next, chop the onions and apple but don't peel the skin. Then, heat the olive oil in a wok and add all the ingredients. Stir-fry till cooked.

****

14) SMOOTHIES
Smoothies are great for constipation as they're easy for the body to digest and are high in fibre. But of course, you'll need a smoothie maker, a blender or something like a magic bullet to make them.

I'm a recent convert to smoothies and initially wasn't sure what ingredients to use. Although there are thousands of recipes on the Web, I decided to invest time and money in experimenting to discover what I liked. So, I did a supermarket shop and bought lots of fruit and vegetables, seeds, nut milk, and flavoured sparkling water. Then I spent a few hours making small smoothies, mixing and matching the ingredients, and tasting them till I came up with my preference. Although it took some time and a little money, I would recommend doing this, as I never make a smoothie I dislike and then pour it down the drain.

Here's a summary of what I discovered, but I want to stress these are my preferences; yours may be different.

o Bananas and avocados thicken the smoothie; my preference was for avocados.
o The flavour of dates, figs, prunes, bananas, and oranges was overpowering for me.
o Apples and pears tasted good, but I wasn't sure if I liked the smoothie's texture; my preference was for berries, especially raspberries. I also like kiwi, and when they're in season, I add them to my smoothie.
o I didn't see the benefit of adding dried fruit such as sultanas and raisins, especially as they're high in calories.
o I didn't like the taste of flaxseeds/linseeds in the smoothie, but chia seeds were excellent with no taste.
o For liquids, I tried almond milk, soy milk, coconut drink, flavoured water, sparkling water, and fruit juice - the coconut drink was my favorite.
o I decided against adding vegetables like spinach, kale, or celery, preferring a sweet smoothie.

So, I decided on coconut drink (not coconut milk), berries, avocado, and chia seeds. Then, I came up with the recipe below, which I love and make often.

LOW-CARB RASPBERRY SMOOTHIE
Total 10g fibre and 4.3g carbs per serving.

Ingredients
250ml/1 cup coconut drink, fibre 0.1g and carbs 1g
60g/2oz raspberries, fibre 3.9g and carbs 2.5g
½ tbsp/6.5g chia seeds, fibre 2g and carbs 0.7g
60g/2oz avocado, fibre 4g and carbs 1.1g
½ tsp sweetener (optional)

As I use frozen avocado and raspberries, I prepare the smoothie 30 minutes before drinking to allow the ingredients to defrost. This also pre-soaks the chia seeds, which is beneficial. The seeds form a mucilaginous gel with the liquid, making it easier to digest and helps soothe inflamed tissue in the gut lining.

Frozen berries and avocado chunks can be bought all year round and stored in the freezer, so there's no waste. You can replace the coconut drink with a liquid of your choice and raspberries with any berry. If you don't like a cold smoothie, pop it in the microwave for 10/20 seconds to take the chill off, although I wouldn't do it for longer as it may destroy the nutrients in the ingredients.

FERMENTED SMOOTHIE
Use the Raspberry Smoothie recipe but replace ½ cup of the liquid with goat's milk Kefir, and you can also add 30g/1oz

sauerkraut. Berries have a strong flavour and will mask the taste of the Kefir or sauerkraut. Kefir can have a powerful effect on the body, so start with half a cup. For goat's milk Kefir and sauerkraut, see recipes 22 and 23.

****

15) BARMBRACK (IRISH TEA LOAF) OR TWELVE FRUIT MUFFINS

Total 27.5g of fibre in the whole loaf and 2.3g per muffin.

For the Barmbrack, use a loaf tin 8½ x 4½ (21 x 11.5cm).

For the muffins use a 12-cup (large cups) baking tray.

Bake the loaf for 60 minutes and the muffins for 20 minutes.

Bake at oven temperature:

Gas 4 / 350°F / 180°C / fan oven 160°C

Ingredients

300g/10oz dried fruit of choice, fibre 5g

240ml/8oz tea bag and hot water

*240g/8oz wholemeal raising flour, fibre 22.5g

1 large egg

2 level tbsp powdered sweetener

OR

75g/2.5oz brown sugar

*When using plain flour, add 1 teaspoon of baking powder.

Make the tea with the hot water and teabag in a measuring jug. Take the teabag out and top up the liquid if it's reduced. Put the dried fruit and tea into a bowl and leave to soak while mixing the other ingredients. You can also soak the fruit for one hour or overnight to make the loaf more flavoured. Place the flour, powdered sweetener, or sugar into a bowl and mix. Next, add the dried fruit and tea mixture and the whisked egg. If the mixture is dry, add one half or one whole egg. Mix well. Put the mixture in the loaf tin or the 12-cup baking tray. Once cooked, store the sliced loaf or muffins in an airtight container.

NOTE: to freeze, first put individual slices or muffins on a tray in the freezer till frozen, then put them in one freezer bag. By freezing first, they won't stick together. To defrost, put a slice of Barmbrack or a muffin in a paper towel and microwave on high for 30 seconds.
****

16) ALL-BRAN LOAF
Makes 10 slices.
Total 35g fibre for the whole loaf or 3.5g per slice.
NOTE: soak the dried fruit for 10 minutes before starting. Some of the mixture is left to soak for one hour.

Ingredients
120g/4oz All Bran cereal, fibre 32.4g
120g/4oz caster sugar or 2 to 3 tbsp powdered sweetener
120g/4oz sultanas, fibre 2.6g
½ cup tea
300ml/10oz milk of choice
*120g/4oz plain white flour
1 teaspoon baking powder
*Wholemeal flour can increase the fibre, but it makes a denser loaf.

Bake for one hour at oven temperature:
Gas 3 / 325°F / 160°C / fan oven 140°C.

Before starting, soak the dried fruit in 1/2 cup of hot tea for 10 minutes but do not strain the tea. Next, add all the ingredients except the flour and baking powder into a large mixing bowl and leave to soak for at least one hour. Then, mix the flour and baking powder and fold them into the mixture. Do not overmix, or the cake will be tough. Pour the mixture into a greased loaf tin, approximate inside measurements 21cm x 11.5cm (8.½" x 4½"). Allow the loaf to cool in the baking tin, then turn it onto a cooling rack. When cool, cut into ten slices and store in an airtight container.

NOTE: to freeze, put individual slices on a tray in the freezer until frozen, then put them in one freezer bag. By freezing first, they won't stick together. To defrost, place a slice of the loaf in a paper towel and microwave on high for 30 seconds.
****

17) EIGHT LOW-CARB SWEET FLAXSEED BISCUITS
Total 3.4g of fibre and 0.2g of carbs per biscuit.

Ingredients
100g/3.5oz ground flaxseed, fibre 27.3g and 0.6g carbs
1 large egg, fibre 0g and 0.4g carbs
1.5 tbsp powdered sweetener
Bake for 15 minutes at oven temperature:
Gas 4 / 350°F / 180°C / fan oven 160°C

Break the egg into a cup and whisk slightly. Add sweetener to the flaxseed and mix. Add the egg and mix till combined. Divide the mixture into eight portions. Flatten each piece with your hand and shape it into a circle. Or, as an easy alternative, press the flaxseed mixture into a 20cm/8" square baking tin. Cut the mixture with a knife into eight rectangles, then bake as usual. Once cooled, put the biscuits in an airtight container. Store this in the fridge as the flaxseeds can become mouldy.

NOTE: if you prefer a savory biscuit, omit the sugar, and add grated cheese, finely chopped onion, or chives.
****

18) DESSERTS OR SNACKS FOR ONE
Mix and match some of the ingredients below to make a delicious high-fibre dessert or snack. Use fresh or frozen avocado, berries, and apple slices. Put a portion of one of the fruits into a bowl, and if desired, sprinkle with sweetener and flaxseeds. Top with a bit of cream or a non-dairy cream replacement. Chia seeds should be soaked in water for 20 minutes before serving; if it's too thick, add some milk to thin it.

Ingredients
60g/2oz chopped avocado, fibre 4g and carbs 0.9g
60g/2oz raspberries, fibre 3.9g and carbs 2.5g
120g/4oz *chopped apple, fibre 2.7g and carbs 13.4g
120g/4oz rhubarb, fibre 2.2g and carbs 5.4g
1 tbsp/8g ground flaxseed, fibre 2.2g and carbs 0.4g
1 tsp/4g chia seeds, fibre 1.2g and carbs 0.4g
*You can microwave the apple to soften it.
****

19) LOW-CARB RHUBARB CRUMBLE FOR TWO

One serving has 4.8g of fibre and 5.8g of carbs.

<u>Ingredients</u>
210g/7oz frozen rhubarb, fibre 3.6g and carbs 5.4g
1-2 tsp sweetener
30g/1oz almond flour, fibre 1.9g and carbs 2.1g
15g/½oz flaxseeds, fibre 4.1g and carbs 0.2g
1 tbsp sweetener
1 tbsp butter

Bake for 25 minutes at oven temperature:
Gas 6 / 400°F / 200°C / fan oven 180°C.
Microwave the rhubarb in a bowl with one to two teaspoons of sweetener. Put the rhubarb in an ovenproof dish. Next, mix the almond flour, flaxseeds, and 1 tbsp sweetener in a bowl. Add the butter to the mixture and mix with your hands till it's like thick breadcrumbs. Top the rhubarb with the crumble and bake in the oven.
****

20) LOW-CARB COCOA DRINK FOR ONE

Total 0.9g fibre and 0.6g of carbs per serving.

<u>Ingredients</u>
1 tsp/3g cocoa powder, fibre 0.8g and carbs 0.3g
1 cup/250ml almond milk, fibre 1g and carbs zero
1 tbsp/15ml single cream, carbs 0.3g
Sweetener
Mix the cocoa with a bit of milk to form into a paste in a large mug. Add everything else, stir and microwave till hot.

If you don't eat dairy, then use a non-dairy cream replacement.
****

21) GOAT'S MILK KEFIR

Kefir is a fermented milk drink, like a thin yogurt made by soaking Kefir grains (a type of culture) in milk. You can purchase Kefir grains on the Web. They look like small rubbery cauliflower pieces. Here are simple instructions to give you an idea of how to make Kefir. The Facebook group *Kefir* has 30,000 members and has all the information and support you need.

Place one teaspoon of Kefir grains in a glass jar and top with one cup of full-fat milk. Use goat's milk, as casein the protein in cow's milk, can be constipating. Place the lid on the jar and leave it in a cupboard to ferment for 24 hours. The Kefir is then strained, poured back into the glass jar, and stored in the refrigerator till used. The grains will multiply, and you can then add more milk.

The grains are either used again or put in a small container covered with some milk in the fridge.
****

22) EASY-PEASY SAUERKRAUT

For information and support on making fermented food join the Facebook Group *Fermenting: Healing Through Food* or check out YouTube videos on making sauerkraut.

Ingredients

2.2lb/1kg fresh cabbage or an easy alternative is a bag of frozen, chopped cabbage (defrost first before using)
2 tbsp of salt, either Celtic or Pink Himalayan

If using fresh cabbage, cut it into thin strips. Then, use the frozen cabbage as it is in the bag but defrosted. Put the cabbage in a large bowl. Add the salt and massage with both hands for 5 minutes, let it rest for 5 minutes, then massage again for 5 minutes. Next, squeeze out as much liquid as possible and put the cabbage into a one litre glass jar. Pour the brine into the jar and ensure the cabbage is under the brine, or mould will form. A space of 2.54cm/1" needs to be above the brine. Put the lid tightly on the jar and place it in a warm cupboard for at least ten days to allow the sauerkraut to ferment.

NOTE: I use a Lakeland fermentation jar with an air-release valve. It comes in two sizes 1 litre or 1.4 litres.
****

Dear Reader

I hope you've enjoyed reading *It's All About The Food*, and it's given you some ideas on changes to make to your diet that may help you poop more regularly.

Blessings!
Helen

Printed in Great Britain
by Amazon

84413087R00108